The WISDÖM YEARS

UNLEASHING your POTENTIAL in LATER LIFE

ZVI LANIR, PHD

Emotional Inheritance

AN IMPRINT OF EXISLE PUBLISHING

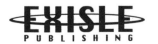

Zvi Lanir, PhD, is the founding president of the Praxis Institute, which, for over 30 years, has specialized in various aspects of coping with disruptive change in personal, social, economic and strategic domains. During the past fifteen years, Dr Lanir has conducted interdisciplinary research to reveal the gaps between the common knowledge on aging and the new opportunities for living our advanced years differently. Dr Zvi Lanir is a graduate of the Israel Defense Forces' Command and Staff College. He has a PhD from the Hebrew University of Jerusalem and has been a visiting scholar at New York's Columbia University.

To Rachel, the mother of my children,
and to Ori, Tamar and Shai — my children.
I only wish that during your childhood
I had known what I know
now that I have embarked on the wisdom years.

First published 2019
Emotional Inheritance
An imprint of Exisle Publishing Pty Ltd
PO Box 864, Chatswood, NSW 2057, Australia
226 High Street, Dunedin, 9016, New Zealand
www.exislepublishing.com

A CiP record for this book is available from the National Library of Australia.

ISBN 978-1-925820-23-2

Designed by Nada Backovic
Cover background image: Shutterstock
Internal images: Zvi Lanir and iStock
Typeset in ITC New Baskerville 9/12pt
Printed in China

This book uses paper sourced under ISO 14001 guidelines from well-managed forests and other controlled sources.

10 9 8 7 6 5 4 3 2 1

An earlier edition of this book was published in Hebrew as T*he Age of Wisdom — The New Age in Human Life,* by Niv Publishing in 1977.

With thanks to Achsah Weinberg for the translation from Hebrew to English.

Disclaimer

While this book is intended as a general information resource and all care has been taken in compiling the contents, neither the author nor the publisher and their distributors can be held responsible for any loss, claim or action that may arise from reliance on the information contained in this book. As each person and situation is unique, it is the responsibility of the reader to consult a qualified professional regarding their personal care.

In the book of life,
the answers aren't in the back.
CHARLIE BROWN

Table of Contents

Preface — Welcome to the Hidden Age   1

Part One — From the Hidden Age to the Wisdom Years   **7**

Chapter 1 — Seeking a New Model of Aging   9

Chapter 2 — Facing up to Retirement: Voices from the Street   15

Chapter 3 — What Can Economics and Demography Tell Us?   31

Chapter 4 — Asking the Experts: The Ladder Paradigm of Aging   39

Chapter 5 — The Evolution of the Aging Brain   49

Chapter 6 — Creating New 'Mind Maps'   63

Chapter 7 — The Age of Wisdom: A New Phase of Life   71

Chapter 8 — The First Hurdle: Ageism   79

**Part Two — Towards a Theory of the
Wisdom Years**   **91**

Chapter 9 — Understanding the Psychological
    Foundations of the Wisdom Years   93

Chapter 10 — How our Brains Work: The
    Challenges Ahead   103

Chapter 11 — Renewing Mind and Body in
    Later Life   115

Part Three — Enjoying the Wisdom Years   **129**

Introduction to Part Three   131

Chapter 12 — Mind Your Body   133

Chapter 13 — Harnessing Our Brain Power   147

Chapter 14 — Finding Happiness and Tackling
    Depression   159

Chapter 15 — Resetting Relationships   171

Chapter 16 — Delaying Old Age   193

Chapter 17 — My Personal Journey   207

References   223
Index   233

Preface

Welcome to the Hidden Age

This book describes my personal experience of the 'hidden age'. At the same time, it's your story as well, whether you've reached it yet or not.

Just a generation ago there was no such thing as a 'hidden age'. The date of birth registered on our personal ID indicated our real age. When our parents reached retirement, they moved from adulthood to old age, literally and figuratively. They accepted the 'old' label imposed by society and started looking old, acting old and feeling old.

However, when I reached my official retirement date, I found it hard to see myself as having reached old age. I felt different. Not like my parents' generation. I didn't feel old, I didn't look old, nor was I ready to be regarded as old. It wasn't just a case of injured dignity — it simply wasn't true. While I was ready to admit that I was no longer young, I wasn't ready to concede that I was old. Oddly, I felt that my true age was a mystery to me. Not yet old, but no longer young — what was I, then?

This mystery of my 'hidden age' intrigued me, and I devoted a lot of time to trying to think it through. While doing so, a host of issues were clamouring for my attention. I started noting these thoughts down on paper, in longhand, to ensure that nothing important was forgotten. As my notes accumulated, I discovered that the subject was far broader and more significant than I had originally assumed.

As I proceeded step by step, it became clear that the issues posed by the 'hidden age' are universally applicable. They shed light on a wholly new social phenomenon, one which we all must face.

While it is directly related to the dramatic increase in life expectancy enjoyed by this generation, in itself this is insufficient to explain the human potential associated with this phenomenon. This dramatic rise in life expectancy carries with it far more than just a quantitative leap in our length of life. Rather, I believe that, in the 21st century, it is giving rise to a new phase of human life — the 'age of wisdom' or the 'wisdom years'. This new period is qualitatively different from adulthood which precedes it, as well as from old age.

As we transition out of adulthood, this age of wisdom enables us to experience a new period of active life, one that is wiser, more balanced and more rewarding than adulthood. In turn, this stage may enable us to postpone many of the negative symptoms of aging to the end of life.

We have received a gift — the gift of the wisdom years. We have not yet understood it, nor discovered how to live it. In this book, I seek to reveal the bounty hidden within this unexpected gift.

I entered the age of wisdom in 2004. Since then, I have constantly been experiencing its gifts, while implementing the insights I've been privileged to learn.

At first, my own personal journey was a surprise to me. However, as it unfolded, the journey revealed itself as a process of personal empowerment, discoveries and intriguing implications. This enabled me to challenge the commonly held belief that the official retirement age is inevitably the beginning of old age. I am finding that what I call my 'functional age' is far more important than my chronological age. My functional age reflects my physical, intellectual, mental and social abilities, and determines my quality of life as well as my life expectancy. As I focused on enhancing my functional age, I turned it into a period of personal growth, despite the inevitable toll taken by the biological aging process.

This book is divided into three parts. The first — 'From the Hidden Age to the Wisdom Years' — documents my own journey discovering the essence of this new phase of life and the opportunities it presents. In the second part — 'Towards a Theory of the Wisdom Years' — I set out the theoretical foundations of the subject from the psychological, neurological and biological perspectives. Based on this theory, in the final section of the book — 'Enjoying the Wisdom Years' — I explain how readers can experience this new stage of life for themselves and achieve its potential to the full.

While this book is mainly directed at adults of any age, whom I hope will be inspired to shape their own futures, at the same time it offers new perspectives for professionals who deal with aging. People at or near retirement age will find it immediately relevant as they ponder their future and seek new meaning for their lives. Younger adults may well be encouraged to begin planning their personal future well in advance. In addition, I hope that academics and health professionals will be inspired to devise new ways of planning and caring for communities who are poised to enter the wisdom years.

The aim of this book is to better understand life — not necessarily to contribute to science. While it is based on a wide spectrum of scientific data, I've chosen not to overload it with the detailed references associated with academic discourse.

If you, the reader, use this book for academic purposes only, I've failed in my task as author. On the other hand, if it is used purely as a manual, I haven't achieved my purpose either. Theory and practice complement each other in the story of my journey — a journey that each of us can embark on — as my personal experiences and insights clarify and enrich what science teaches us.

I would like you to find yourself in this book as you search for and ponder new possibilities in your life. I hope that my story will encourage you to start your own personal voyage of discovery as you journey towards your own wisdom years.

PART ONE

From the Hidden Age
to the Wisdom Years

Chapter 1

Seeking a New Model of Aging

It all started in 2004, on the day I received a formal letter from the Department of Social Security, informing me that I had become eligible for the old age pension. Sceptical, I read the letter several times. Me? Old!? At the time, I felt I was in my prime, enjoying an active and vibrant life — but now someone else was presuming to tell me I was old.

I felt something was very wrong with the situation. True — I was no longer young, but at the same time I most definitely did not feel old. The term 'old' did not reflect my essential sense of myself, nor the stage of life which I had reached. My reflections produced a question that sounded distinctly weird, even to myself: So what am I?

My reaction to the government's letter can be clarified by understanding a little about my background. I am founder and owner of the Praxis Research Institute, an independent research organization established during the last decade of the twentieth century. At Praxis we specialize in identifying 'perceptual relevance' gaps, which are triggered by fundamental — but poorly understood — changes in the human environment. Such gaps occur because people tend to use familiar tools to cope with social, cultural and technological change, rather than developing new perceptions and coping methods.[1]

The 21st century is characterized by a constant stream of concurrent, rapid, fundamental changes — more than humanity has ever previously encountered. In the past, transformative changes, such as the discovery of fire, the invention of the wheel and the printing press, and the Industrial Revolution, were infrequent and slow in their implementation. Nowadays, we experience numerous, concurrent, life-altering changes, which affect us far more rapidly and which occur on a large scale. Revolutions in the fields of computing, automation, social media, Big Data and autonomous vehicles impact us daily; however, we are not yet equipped to fully understand the opportunities they present or the dangers they pose.

I specialize in assisting people and organizations identify the perceptual relevance gaps which they are experiencing as they relate to a new reality — the major role of Praxis. In addition, we help shape new perceptions and action methods to help manage these new situations. Thus, when I received the 'old age' letter from Social Security, I immediately recognized that I was facing the kind of situation I train others to deal with. While no longer young, I do not consider myself old. So what am I?

The Social Security document stated that for an Israeli male, 67 is the formal retirement age.[2] However, I wasn't ready to reconcile this message with my life at the time, whether mentally, physically or functionally. Such a categorization may have been relevant for previous generations, but it certainly isn't to mine; it may have suited my grandfather, but it does not fit with the person I am.

So, what then was my 'real' age? The question engendered a sense of mystery. The answer seemed to be an unknown variable within an equally unknown equation.

This discovery produced a distinctive feeling that I have elsewhere called 'fundamental surprise'[3] — an unexpected dramatic event or crisis, highlighting the inadequacy of familiar mindsets for dealing with a newly emergent reality.

One reaction which characterizes almost all 'fundamental surprise' events is denial. Denial manifests as our attempts to explain away new phenomena simply as changes in form or style which require only minor modifications to existing paradigms. It is expressed as dismissal or avoidance of the profound changes needed in the wake of the 'fundamental surprise'. This in turn triggers ongoing and serious crises, as well as the wasting of resources and an increase in human suffering. A long and arduous journey is required to learn the basic lessons needed to cope with such eventualities.

The letter made me realize that I needed to formulate a new mindset, one which would help me to make sense of what I had sensed, but not yet understood. I realized that I had to reframe my own mindset into one that would be a reliable guide for this new phase of my life. Failure to do so would force me to acquiesce in the conventional perceptions of retirement and aging.

I saw that I would have to reframe my whole conceptual system so as to effectively navigate the new reality of my life. I understood that I had to define a new 'narrative identity'[4] for myself, rather than the 'elderly' identity offered by society. This would enable me to view the next phase of my life as a new vista rather than as my exit cue.

As an expert in this field, I've been 'reframing' change for many years, though always for other people. Now I had to put myself through the same process. In any field of expertise, it's easier to deal with others than with yourself. It's even harder when you must change your own engrained conceptions and beliefs.

From the very beginning I realized that this would be a long journey, full of surprises and new insights about the world we live in. I had no idea just how long or fascinating it would turn out to be.

To get an idea of the journey I undertook, I invite you to imagine yourself travelling in an unknown land, without maps, without navigation software and without knowing your goal. Rather like a treasure hunt, at each stop you must find and decipher the clue which will lead you to the next step. I had to learn as I went along, using my acquired knowledge and insights to light the way.

Chapter 2

Facing up to Retirement: Voices from the Street

To begin my journey, I felt that the most logical step was to talk to the people around me who had already retired and find out if they too had an inkling of the 'hidden age'.

I invested a good deal of time trying to find and talk to such people. Whether I had known them before, whether I met them through friends or whether I encountered them sitting on a park bench, I always tried to engage them in conversation about their present life.

Having been part of many such discussions, I was surprised to discover the diversity of solutions to the question 'What will I do with myself?' which people find for themselves when they reach retirement age. I believe that sharing their stories will strike a powerful chord with readers — and remind you of people you know.

I was introduced to Orin,[1] who had just turned 68, by a mutual friend who thought I might be able to help ease his depression. He had recently retired, after a long and flourishing career as a bank branch manager. A wealthy man, he has a loving family of two children and several grandchildren, and is in relatively good health.

For him, aging is not the problem. He does not feel old, nor does he worry about growing old. Rather, his depression is a result of a loss of meaning and passion in his life, and the erosion of his self-esteem — all of which occurred following his retirement.

Orin described his feelings to me in a very vivid manner: 'Just a very short time ago I was wanted and appreciated. Nowadays nobody calls me, and my diary is empty.' He continued: 'My wife scolds me, saying that I annoy her hanging around the house all the time. She says I should get out into the world and find myself again. She's right, of course, but I have no idea how to actually do it.'

I tried to explain to Orin that in order to restore passion and meaning to his life, he needed to distance himself from his professional self-image and formulate a new identity for himself, but without success.

During his entire adult working life, Orin's focus had been on the outside world. He had functioned well when acting according to other people's definitions of his job description. Now Orin needed to shift his focus to his own needs by reframing his thinking, attitudes and behaviour. This task requires a new approach to life, as well as new skills and know-how, changes for which he is ill prepared.

For me, the 'hidden age' was a puzzle calling out to be solved; for Orin, it was a barrier which he didn't know how to overcome.

❊

Reenie, whom I met at the medical clinic, was happy to talk to me while we were waiting our turn to be seen.

She had worked in a bank for her entire adult life, loving the job which kept her on a first-name basis with her long-term clients. Reenie regarded them as friends and felt that they too thought of her as their friend. Only when she retired did she fully understand how much they had meant to her.

Now Reenie feels very lonely, with no one to talk to. She lives alone. She was used to keeping busy by devoting most of her time to her family. She was proud of the babysitting duties she had done for her two granddaughters. She told herself, and anyone who cared to listen, that she had done it to enable her only daughter and son-in-law to develop their careers.

This situation was ideal for Reenie, who loved the time she got to spend with her granddaughters. However, this domestic idyll was shattered when her daughter and son-in-law relocated after receiving a lucrative offer from a prestigious university in the US. She told me that all that remains of her family time are the few moments when she can see her granddaughters on Skype, something which she tries to do every day. Other than that, she has nothing to fill her days and ease her loneliness.

Until her family left, Reenie had been quite healthy; however, since then, she has spent many hours in various medical clinics. Since the doctors have failed to find what's really ailing her, they keep prescribing more and more tests — to rule out specific physical disorders as the cause of her tiredness and depression. She told me that the family physician always ends his consultations by suggesting that she take food supplements, sleep medication and antidepressants. The doctor said that, while these may help, they wouldn't do her any harm.

While we were talking, I noticed that Reenie's clothes were totally out of fashion. I asked her bluntly whether she had bought any new clothes lately. She responded that she'd lost her interest in shopping a long time ago and was happy with the old things she owned. Although she was only 62, she had reconciled herself to being old, dressed like an old lady, and looked old and felt old.

✳

I met Jack in a Barcelona bar. He had sat down next to me at the crowded counter and, without knowing who I was, ordered a drink for me as well as for himself and his date and struck up a conversation in Hebrew. He explained that he had immediately identified me as Israeli, and we became 'friends' after the second drink.

Jack was clearly trying to hide his advancing age. His hair was obviously dyed, his broad gold necklace failed to hide the sagging skin on his neck and he was wearing too much cologne. To complete the somewhat pathetic image, he had his arm around the waist of a good-looking woman who was far younger than him.

Having overheard that I was interested in discussing retirement and aging, he responded in a disparagingly jovial manner and proceeded to tell me what he had been doing since his retirement. To Jack, retirement was like being let out of prison — freed from the restrictions which had surrounded him during his adult life. Not only did he sell his business, but he had also divorced his wife and started dating young women like his current companion. He spent all his money on 'having a good time' as he'd never done before. Retirement for him was a return to the carefree years of being a young bachelor.

Having reiterated the fact that he was 'having a good time', he wished me the same as we parted, rather than the 'keep well' which I normally receive from people my age. I couldn't help contrast Reenie and Jack, who seemed to be going in opposite directions: Reenie had fast-forwarded to old age, while Jack was working hard to turn back the clock.

❄

I met Nate on the street, near a high rise which was being built near my home. We both found ourselves staring at the construction cranes as they lifted heavy loads into the sky. Again, he was the one who initiated the conversation by asking me why I was taking an interest in the cranes. He immediately added that he had been a crane operator, that he missed them as a retiree and that he liked to watch them at work. Nate continued by telling me that when he was employed, he couldn't wait for retirement, as the hard physical work had been wearing him out and getting more and more difficult. He couldn't wait to retire, to finally rest up and 'have some fun'. He had celebrated his retirement by taking a long trip abroad with his wife, something which they had both fantasized about for years. After this initial period of vacation and relaxation, he found he no longer had any reason for getting up in the morning and had started to feel bored.

At first, Nate tried to fend off the boredom by meeting friends or going to malls. Hobbies did not fill the vacuum, either. Nate felt that he was losing his desire to get up in the morning. And why should he get up? The simple happiness he had taken for granted when working as a crane operator had now been lost, and he had no idea how to get it back. He simply missed his cranes!

A few months later, I met Nate on the street again and this time his happiness was obvious. He told me that he was working as a crane operator again. Apparently, his former boss had offered him his job back on a temporary basis, in response to the shortage of operators. Temporarily or not, Nate is happy again.

I was intrigued by the older security guard standing at the main entrance to one of the bank's major branches, checking people as they were about to go in. It was the end of the business day, when customers flock to the bank after finishing work.

It is quite common to find retirees working as security guards. However, this man stood out as he was immaculately dressed and groomed. After opening the door for me with a big smile, and while checking my bag, he asked if he could help by directing me to the line which would best serve my needs.

When I finished what I had to do at the bank I went up to him and thanked him for his help. He responded by saying that since he already knew the bank's 'regulars', he hadn't recognized me, which was why he had offered his help.

Since he had piqued my curiosity, and being the end of his shift, I invited him to join me for coffee at the neighbouring coffee shop. As we sat and talked, he told me the story of his life. He had worked at one of Israel's largest factories his whole life, and had slowly made his way up the company ladder. When he had retired two years ago, his last position had been director of operations.

'Our problem is that since our combined pensions are quite modest,' he said, 'my wife and I need more money to make ends meet. I had dreamed of starting a small business of my own, so I could make money as a freelancer in my specialty. It didn't take me long to realize that after working as a salaried employee for so many years, it was too hard to become self-employed. I wasn't cut out to be my own CEO, my own CFL, and my own sales manager. To succeed as a freelancer, you must learn to sell not only your skills, but yourself as well, and I'd never learned how to do that.'

'The company I'd worked for paid for a short retirement preparation class,' he continued. 'However, it was not enough to properly prepare me for my retirement and the changes I needed to make. After six months of trying to make a go of the business,

I realized that it wasn't going anywhere. I started searching for a job — any job — just so I could bring some money in. So, when I was offered the security guard position, I accepted it. I try my best to preserve my dignity and seek out the more interesting aspects of the job, even though it could be extremely boring and demeaning if you're not a people person.'

I met Eric and Lara when they moved into the apartment building where I live in a quiet area of Tel Aviv, shortly after they had retired. Originally from Haifa, they seemed a well-to-do couple and owned a large apartment with a beautiful view there. Eric had owned his own company, while Lara lectured in sociology. In preparation for retirement, they had purchased a small but centrally located apartment in Tel Aviv, enabling them to take advantage of what the big city could offer them as a retired couple.

As we became friends, I found that Eric and Lara were an intelligent and interesting couple. I was in awe of their zest for living as they immersed themselves in the city's cultural life, taking advantage of what it had to offer and savouring their new experiences. To me, they represented older people who know how to enjoy themselves and make the most of the new period of life which has opened up for them.

After several happy and active years, Lara's health sharply deteriorated and her doctors advised that she needed ongoing supervision and help. Eric and Lara had well-off sons who could have taken them into their own spacious apartments. However, they chose to move to a luxury assisted-living complex out of town.

I continued to visit them at their new home in the assisted-living complex, which offered residents every comfort that older people could desire.

During the conversations we had following their move, they kept trying to convince me — and perhaps themselves, as well — how well they were doing in their new home. Unfortunately, without them admitting it — or even without noticing it — the assisted-living complex had become, for them, a self-contained bubble. Their new way of life meant that they had removed themselves from the multi-generational neighbourhoods they used to live in, places which had provided them with ongoing stimulation and novelty. In their new quarters, they found themselves confined within a group of self-absorbed old men and women whose conversations were mostly about their various ailments and complaints.

Within assisted-living settings, the residents' schedule is usually determined by the management, who decides the activities required to keep them entertained and healthy. In my opinion, such an environment severely limits the scope of the residents' own initiative, with negative impacts on who they are as people. It seemed to me that Eric and Lara had lost their alertness, openness and curiosity, and were accommodating themselves to an ever-narrowing world of 'old people' and comfortable aging.

As I wrote down the stories I had heard, it became clear how varied they were. Each one represents a unique mix of personal background, circumstances, abilities, economic situation, social status, emotions, wishes and a multitude of other intertwined factors.

My first concern was that my analysis and conclusions about other people should not be based on my own situation. I was reminded of the wise saying of Margaret Mead, the famous anthropologist:

'Always remember that you are absolutely unique. Just like everyone else.' The information I had collected represented personal, individual biographies. Each person on earth is marked by a unique combination of options and desires, and I could not hope to account for them all.

However, beyond this incredible variety, I noticed that the question which dominated my thoughts — the issue of the 'hidden age' — simply had not occurred to any of the people I had talked to. They carried on with their lives after retirement without giving a thought to what it meant. There were those seeking to make the most of what was available to them, others who sought to escape back to a younger life and those who skipped forward to old age — each in her or his own way.

All the retirees I had talked to had sought to deal with their new situation by responding to the issues which faced them as they cropped up. It occurred to none of them to try to understand this new, hidden age that they had entered in a global or abstract manner, nor how it might affect their current lives or their futures.

Redefining the Problem

It became clear that I had made a mistake by expecting these encounters to provide responses to the issues which so occupied my thoughts.

A different focus was needed. If I was setting out to understand the current transportation crisis, it wouldn't make sense to do so by acquainting myself with the various models of cars on the road. A 'fundamental crisis'[2] of this kind must be analyzed and understood on a much more abstract level. Only once the essential character of the phenomenon has been understood can one explore solutions to the more immediate and visible problems posed by the crisis. I had learned this lesson when dealing with other fundamental crises; I now needed to apply my experience to the one on the table.

This, then, was the new goal I had to set when seeking the next step in my journey of understanding.

The transportation crisis at least includes the term 'transportation' as a key to what I have elsewhere called its methodological conceptualization. However, the conceptual key that might unlock the 'hidden age' was still missing.[3]

I decided to try the internet. With a single key click I found myself swamped with data on the biological aspects of aging — graying hair, rougher skin, weakening muscles, lowered calcium, and so on. I also found a plethora of information on 'aging illnesses' — loss of memory, vision and hearing impairments and — the worst threat of all — the various types of dementia. I also found many suggestions for deferring these symptoms as long as possible.

The same went for retirement: I found a lot of sites and articles dealing with retirement, with the pension crisis triggered by the sharp rise in life expectancy, and numerous suggestions on how to cope with these issues.

I also found sites dedicated to what is often called 'the golden age', discussing the entertainment and social needs of people who have already retired. These sites reflect the attempt to provide retirees with 'golden age' clubs — groups for those evicted from the clubs of adulthood.

Libraries and bookstores also offer a wide range of popular literature giving advice on how to prepare for retirement and live well in old age.

But as neither the internet nor the books I found dealt with the 'hidden age' or the issues surrounding it, I was forced to widen the scope of my search. My next step would be to investigate what the sciences of economics and demography could teach me about the implications of our dramatic rise in life expectancy.

Chapter 3

What Can Economics and Demography Tell Us?

Over the past century, human life expectancy has risen by around 30 years. This rate is not showing any signs of slowing down. Two world wars, the 1918 influenza epidemic, the AIDS epidemic (which started towards the end of the twentieth century) and even the uncontrolled growth of the world's crowded megacities do not seem to have affected this demographic trend.

This is a novel and unparalleled phenomenon. In evolutionary terms, it represents a mere blink in time. In previous eras, it was exceptional for someone to reach the age of 40. A slight rise in life expectancy became apparent towards the end of the medieval period, but was still minimal by today's standards. Dramatic change started to occur only in the nineteenth century. However, for a person born in 1900 in the US, life expectancy still did not exceed 47.

Since then, the rate of change has been exponential. If our life expectancy bank is imagined as a period of 24 hours, then people today are enjoying an additional six hours. To put it another way, every four years another year is added to our lifespan. In the First World, a person reaching the age of 60 has a life expectancy of close to 90,[1] and their grandchildren's life expectancy is 100.

Modern society is in the process of becoming an aging society. The UN has predicted that by the year 2050 the developed countries will contain around 26 per cent of people aged 65 or older.[2] One out of three citizens will be retired, and around one in ten will be 80 or older. Furthermore, it is anticipated that people 65 or older will outnumber children under five.

As the graph below shows, the population of the developed world is rapidly aging, and the poorer nations are only a few decades behind.

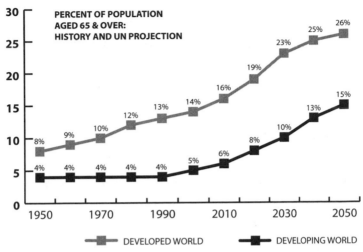

Source: https://www.un.org/en/development/desa/population/
pdf/commission/2007/keynote/chatterj.pdf

We've become used to viewing the age spectrum as a pyramid, with a wide base representing the young which narrows as people's age rises. But this is no longer the case — the pyramid is beginning to invert.

And what of the future? Will our life expectancy rise beyond 100? The experts differ on this question. Some scientists argue that the demographic tsunami is still far from reaching its peak; others claim that it will reach an upper limit beyond which our biological systems will collapse.[3]

So how does this dramatic increase in life expectancy affect the economy, society and individuals?

If we are to believe the economists, the answer is a depressing one. Their basic assumption is that once we retire, we start being old. As long as we were working, we were an economic asset; from then on, we become an ever-growing burden and liability to society.

Based on this assumption, economists predict that the aging of the population will lead to a significant increase in public expenditure on health services, hospitalization and nursing services. The public health system is already poorly resourced in terms of beds, doctors and nurses to serve the current needs of the population. Economists predict that health services will collapse, and that public and private spending for nursing services will escalate.

As a result of our enhanced lifespans, the imbalance between our working and retirement years will mean that, as individuals, we will be unable to accumulate sufficient pension funds to support us through the long years of retirement. Governments will have to face up to this gap, and take action to deal with it. They will be driven to increase the retirement age, despite the political difficulties involved. However, it seems doubtful if this move will cover the shortfall in pension funds experienced by many countries. As a result, taxes will need to be raised and government services curtailed — not just those aimed at the retired sector, but for the general population. In addition, governments will find it difficult to allocate the funds necessary for the creation of new jobs. This in turn will make it harder for the younger generation to fund the increased needs of the elderly.

The economists' predictions are frightening. However, is it inevitable that the aging of society will trigger all these negative results?

As I continued to investigate these questions, I discovered that the economists' calculations are based on a mistaken premise — that the most important figure is a person's chronological age. This assumption ignores the fact that today's 70 year old is not the 70 year old of past generations. Not only do people live longer, but they are healthier, better educated, can take better care of themselves and contribute to society far more than they could in previous generations.

A research project conducted in 2007 compared a contemporary group of 72 year olds to people who were 72 in 1992.[4] It was found that the 2007 cohort performed better, both cognitively and functionally, than their 1990s peers. Mentally, their abilities were comparable to people who were fifteen years younger than them in the previous generation. The saying '70 is the new 50' would seem to be backed up by science.

Our health is certain to deteriorate at some later stage of our lives. However, unlike previous generations, chronic medical conditions are no longer an inevitable pass to the geriatric ward. In many cases, modern medicine allows us to control the chronic diseases of old age, enabling us to continue to function actively and mindfully until the very last phase of our lives.

Twenty-first century conditions require a different approach to calculating life expectancy: taking account of people's physical, mental and social abilities will yield a more accurate picture of their true 'functional age'. Such calculations will provide very different results from those provided by conventional economists, who only take chronological age into account.

As life expectancy continues to rise, the gap between a person's 'chronological age' and their 'functional age' in later life grows wider. We've all had the experience of meeting 60 year olds who act as though they are already elderly, while some folk in their 80s are more active and vibrant than most of our younger acquaintances. The older people are, the greater the potential disparity between their chronological age and their functional age.

In face of this evidence, I had to wonder why economists continue to ignore it. It seems to be just another expression of a phenomenon I've encountered before: the human tendency to interpret facts according to our deeply held preconceptions, to give credence to data which supports these beliefs and undervalue data which refutes them.

Beyond all this, I was troubled by a far more basic reality: In evolutionary terms, it seems that we were created by nature to live only a few years after we complete our biological roles, and after we no longer have the strength to engage in productive activity. However, nowadays we continue living for a long time after we've successfully procreated and the kids have left home — and we certainly don't conveniently 'roll over' following retirement.

So what is the meaning of the extra years we now so commonly enjoy? Do we continue to live just to demonstrate our dwindling capacity for internal growth and contribution to society? Are they to be defined solely as years when we become increasingly dependent on external economic, social and medical support? Are we simply experiencing a slowed-down version of the aging process, compared with previous generations? Is this all that we can hope for?

Demography likewise failed to give me compelling answers to these questions. Akin to economics, it contents itself with tracking changes in population trends without providing a human meaning and content to these changes.

Next, I decided to seek better answers from gerontologists, health-care professionals who specialize in the later years of human life.

Chapter 4

Asking the Experts: The Ladder Paradigm of Aging

What implications does the increase in life expectancy have for retirement? Clearly, the next stop on my journey was gerontology — the study of the social, cultural, psychological, cognitive and biological aspects of aging.

I made a point of studying any material I could find on the subject and attended professional conventions. This allowed me to get to know, talk to and even become friends with some of Israel's most distinguished gerontologists. I learned a lot from them, and gained a true appreciation of the mission of gerontological care. However, despite this, many of the broad questions I had accumulated during my 'hidden age' journey remained unanswered.

It seems to me that academic research on aging has yet to catch up with the rapid qualitative changes which are marking people's later years in the 21st century.

Despite the wealth and variety of opinions in gerontology, as in any professional field, there is a commonly accepted paradigm which no longer seems relevant to the reality of today — a contradiction that has indeed been noted by some gerontologists.[1] Despite this, most practitioners still adhere to the classic gerontological paradigm.

According to this model, a human life can be described in terms of climbing up a ladder, reaching the top and climbing down the other side. During childhood and adulthood, an individual's functional skills keep increasing; this leads step by step to personal advancement, culminating in the achievement of a personal peak. After this, the subject's skills and abilities begin to diminish, again step by step, culminating in old age and death.

In some respects, we already begin losing physical abilities during our twenties. However, in the gerontological model, it is retirement which signals the transition from upward movement on the ladder to the steep decline of the downward leg.

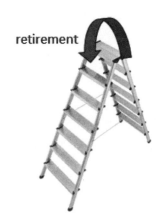

retirement

THE LADDER PARADIGM

Illustration © Zvi Lanir

The recent sharp increase in life expectancy has not invalidated this paradigm in the eyes of gerontology specialists. Rather, the paradigm has been modified so that the rate of decline, or the angle of the ladder, is now viewed as less steep. The decline is still present, but has slowed a little.

According to the revised model, a person's descent on the developmental ladder unfolds over three stages: younger old age (60 to 70), middle old age (70 to 80), and the very old — 80 years and older.

This paradigm, which views the human lifespan in terms of upward and downward progress on our individual ability ladder, has been supported by numerous studies comparing the abilities of older and younger people. Their findings demonstrated many areas in which older people scored lower than the young. However, on re-examination, many of these results have proved questionable. A large proportion of these studies were conducted in retirement and nursing homes, places where people view themselves as old and therefore act old. In such places, gerontologists found what they were looking for, and then applied their conclusions to the general population. Little wonder that their research has generally supported stereotypical views of the elderly.

More recent research, conducted among retired elderly people who continue to live and function within their original physical and social milieux, has offered a more varied and encouraging picture.

Accepting the ladder paradigm at face value ignores a very important question: what are the skills needed for coping in one's later years, and how do they differ from those required when young? The decreased skill set observed in research on older people may simply reflect the reality that they don't need this specific combination of skills to the same extent. The changes in skill sets observed could be explained by an evolution or reorganization of cognitive skills — the very capabilities needed for coping with the new demands and needs of being older, and functioning in a world where people's lives are longer and better. Standardized tests check for skills important to human functioning when young. However, these tests may no longer be relevant for determining function in older subjects.

The conceptual weight of the classic gerontology paradigm may have caused researchers to ignore the possibility that an older person develops other, alternative cognitive skills, which demand a different and higher level of organizational structure in the brain. Given the increase in life expectancy, these new skills may enable older people to keep on enjoying life without becoming 'old'.

Older people employ different processes of thought and logic than younger people, even when coping with the same tasks. For example, in one study, older people were asked to suggest various configurations of model houses set on a lawn. They were also asked whether different configurations would affect the extent of grass to be mowed. Their answers were intriguing, if not objectively correct. Rather than pointing out that the total extent of grass to be mowed would not be affected by different configurations, they indicated that it would be harder to mow many small areas of grass between the houses, as opposed to one large area, and that it would take longer.

In another study, it was found that when subjects were asked to summarize a story they had been told, the attention to detail recorded was qualitatively different between older and younger subjects.[2] The older people in the study paid attention to the metaphorical or moral meanings of the stories — going to a level beyond the bare narrative. They made connections between the information presented and their knowledge of the real world, thereby activating a rich interpretive process. In contrast, the younger subjects, who had answered the same questions, absorbed the information passively and did not relate it to their prior knowledge and experience.

Such examples suggest that older people are not satisfied with factual knowledge and insist on meaning, nor are they willing to ignore practical issues such as how a project might be implemented. In many ways, older people's thinking is more complex than younger people — who often assume that there is always only one 'correct solution'.[3]

The Harvard Project on Aging, an adult developmental study well known for its long duration and broad scope, followed 825 people from their late teen years until they were very old.[4] Some of the subjects lived past their 80s, having been under scrutiny by the project team for over 60 years. The researchers found that the common assumption that one's personal growth stops at 60 is simply wrong.

Initially, the project focused exclusively on eighteen-year-old students who had begun their higher education at the prestigious Harvard University. However, critics pointed out that this sample would be an elitist group with a high IQ, and thus no reliable conclusions could be drawn about the population in general. A new group was therefore added to the study. Young men from poor, crime-ridden neighbourhoods. Most of them were children of immigrants; a quarter had been held back a year in school at least once before they were fourteen. To further diversify the project, a group of women was added — a cohort which had already been under study since the 1920s.

George Vaillant, one of the managers of the Harvard Project, wrote a book about his experiences of working with the study.[5] He was in his 40s when he joined the project, and at the time was mostly interested in middle age. He interviewed the 50-year-old subjects and assumed that he would not find a growth spurt in this group. However, when he interviewed those who were over 70 (in 2000, when 70 per cent of the participants were over 70), he was astounded by the development and progress which they had exhibited since their 50s. He commented: 'The truth is that I didn't know anything … What could I have known? I was only 43.'

The participants were also amazed by the development which they had experienced in their own later years. One remarked: 'We had not previously given any thought to the options presented by our later years: new forms of intimacy coupled with love, opportunities for work, activities with purpose and added values — like learning, knowledge, giving and caring within the community … The ability to view age as a continuous human development requires a revolutionary change of paradigm.'[6]

The Harvard Project, as well as a number of other studies, demonstrates that people who live longer are those who, at an advanced age, have developed new skills of thinking, emotion, action and social involvement. These people succeed in having an active life right up to their death, even when they suffer from malignant diseases.

Nowadays, many gerontologists recognize that aging is not a relentless chronological clock. However, when physicians examine octogenarians whose mental and physical abilities resemble those of 60 year olds, many continue to categorize them as unique.

Contemporary gerontologists are questioning the concepts behind the ladder paradigm. However, as Thomas Kuhn demonstrated in the 1960s, in his book *The Structure of Scientific Revolutions*, such doubts will not necessarily trigger a change in the paradigm.[7] According to Kuhn, even an 'epistemological crisis' (the inability of the current paradigm to provide a satisfactory explanation of new evidence) will not necessarily prompt a shift to a new model. Such a shift cannot be made until a 'sociological crisis' occurs — where a new generation of researchers takes its place in the forefront of the discipline, enabling the acceptance of a new paradigm.

In gerontology, the conventional paradigm is still in transition. It may be many more years before this process changes the social and economic conceptions and practical outcomes which are based on the classic paradigm.

The stereotypes created as a result of the ladder paradigm have influenced social behaviour and governmental policies and actions, which in turn are inextricably linked to a multitude of entrenched institutional and business interests. These ties make it even harder to move away from the social stigmas and practical effects associated with the ladder paradigm.

When assessing what I had learned so far about the revolutionary effects of the increase in human life expectancy, it became clear that, in general, I had gained negative insights — or 'what it isn't'. While the sources of the mistaken assumptions which we take as fact may have become clearer, as well as the stigmas which they project on older people, I had made little progress in getting an answer to the question, 'what is it?'.

However, I gained more positive responses at the next stop on my journey — neurology.

Chapter 5

The Evolution of the Aging Brain

The past few years have seen some major advances in neurological research. Most of these have been facilitated by new technologies which image the brain's activity in real time.

Researchers are now able to view a subject's brain while engaged in a variety of mental activities, an ability which has triggered a dramatic revolution in brain science. The impact of this ongoing revolution can be compared to the effect of the telescope on astronomy or the microscope on medicine.

These new tools have enabled researchers to demonstrate that while some brain functions diminish with advancing age, others improve.[1] The specific skills which decline, as well as those which improve with age, are in the process of being mapped, leading to a deeper understanding of the correlations between them.

The skills which decline include memory, the speed of information processing, the ability to learn new details and the ability to perform concurrent tasks. For many, the decline in the brain's functioning in our advanced years is symbolized by the deterioration of memory, a loss which is often all too obvious. Indeed, in later years we all experience a marked decline in our ability to remember names, numbers and words. I find myself frustrated when, in the middle of a conversation or lecture, I cannot remember this kind of information. Although I don't forget the *meaning* of the word which has 'eluded' my memory, I cannot recall it in real time, at the moment when I need it. The name or word hasn't 'escaped' — it's just hidden somewhere in my brain. It's poised on the tip of my tongue but is refusing to exit.

For example, while my brain recognizes the familiar local store I'm standing in, at the same time I just can't remember the owner's name. While I'm feeling frustrated, my brain finds ways of getting around this problem without him noticing my agitation. Often, when I've been out of the store for a while, busy with something else, the name will just pop up.

We can use modern technology — such as Google, Wikipedia and electronic dictionaries — to get around the challenges which our memories pose when we try unsuccessfully to remember names, numbers, dates and words. I use such tools to remember names which I have not had occasion to use for a while. I've also developed strategies to circumvent uncomfortable situations — for example, when I forget the name of a person I meet or other names which come up in conversation.

During our later years we also experience problems with our short-term memory, also known as our 'working memory'. Not only may we forget where we put our glasses or keys, but we can even end up in a room without remembering why we went there in the first place.

This reduction in short-term memory can also be managed with simple strategies. I make sure to always put my glasses and keys in the same place. Dementia and Alzheimer's disease excepted, research has demonstrated that memory loss in advanced age is not so serious, nor does it have a meaningful impact on day-to-day life. We should not allow this apparent memory loss to depress us — and thus make a minor problem into a major one.

While we may forget names and dates, our brain compensates by providing us with a more precise understanding of the world and the issues that face us. As we age, we become better equipped to ignore unimportant details and to skip unnecessary steps in the thinking and doing process. Our personal store of experience furnishes our minds with intuition, which guides us in our decisions without necessarily having to rely on details.

As we get on in years, our data-processing speed slows down and we find it harder to multitask. This is the reason why the elderly, more than younger people, are prone to accidents while texting and driving. When my grandson suggests that we play computer games which require rapid co-ordination between several concurrent actions, I know that there's not a chance in the world of me beating him. This may be the reason why he so loves playing with me! However, the fact that I'm sure to lose doesn't deter me, and I gladly take up every opportunity of playing with him. The benefits include the opportunity to keep our relationship vibrant; in addition, I get a chance to improve my co-ordination skills, even though I know I'll never catch up to his.

In their later years, people tend to become slower to grasp details, especially technical ones. While some have put this down to the brain being 'tired' or 'lazy' in older people, fMRI testing has found that this is not the case. The older brain does not experience an inevitable decline in function. It is, however, more focused than the younger brain on learning to deal with broader issues rather than absorbing details.

I realized this for myself when I tried to change my Android phone for an iPhone — which would have meant familiarizing myself with a new set of operating procedures. Younger people migrate from one system to another easily, almost intuitively. For me, however, it was difficult, and I found I couldn't manage it. This doesn't mean that my brain is tired or lazy — otherwise I couldn't plan and write this book. What it *does* mean is that my brain is calibrated to a different thought setting.

Transforming our Thinking

Current neurological research suggests that we need to reconsider our interpretation of the transformations occurring in the older brain. Rather than viewing these changes in terms of decline, we should recognize the abilities which come to the forefront as we age, while at the same time we shed skills which may no longer be needed. These new abilities redefine our skill set, which in turn helps us to cope with the reality of our changing needs and the issues they throw up. As we get older, we gain the ability to think these issues through in a new way, considering them in depth and within a broader context.

One explanation for the apparent decline in memory function in the elderly is the differences in the way they approach and process new situations. When faced with a new situation, older people try to relate it to their previous experience, without responding to each detail as a separate entity. For people in my age group, this manifests as a reduced ability to remember words and details, which may explain why we often forget the name of an acquaintance we've met on the street. At the same time, using our new skill set, we may find that we can discover new facts about the person we are talking to — things more important than his or her name. For instance, it may be easier for us to figure out that the other person is lying, since our older brain is able to trigger more associations and connections with our previous life experiences.

As we get older, we rely less on our data-processing abilities and capacity to make fast responses, and more on intuitive processes. This slowing down is meant to enable us to take the time to reflect. When young, our reality required us to process a lot of information simultaneously and react quickly. When we are older, there is less need for these skills, and so we can allow ourselves to have slower reaction times. While the brain's capacity for parallel processing and quick responses may have reduced, our level of maturity means that we can react according to our senses and feelings, as seen through the lenses of reflection and experience.

In studies comparing the speed of data processing and comprehension between younger and older subjects, younger people were indeed faster. However, the older group took into account considerations that were based on personal associations and life experiences, and less on raw data. For example, in one study, two groups were asked to read paragraphs containing unusual words and expressions. While the older subjects were slower to read and process the material, they showed a better understanding of it. They were using distinctive mental processes — which at first glance may seem irrelevant — to acquire a richer understanding of the issues posed in the texts.

In later life, this ability and desire to examine things through multiple lenses explains the common phenomenon of older people appearing to be 'scatterbrained'. They seem to be skipping from one subject to the next, while ignoring the apparent subject of the conversation. When they start talking, it's hard to stop them. They talk ... and talk ... and talk. Their minds seem to be all over the place, and they have a hard time concentrating and keeping to the point. In our later years, we feel the need to examine multiple scenarios and associations around each subject we consider. When this tendency passes a certain point, other people back off. However, when this kind of enquiry is conducted consciously, with intent, it provides a multi-dimensional investigation of the new issues and questions which older people face.

As we age, the way in which we categorize things becomes broader and more sophisticated, and thus we are less dependent on accumulating specific data. In a study analyzing the diagnoses made by older doctors, it was found that their decisions were based less on attempts at comprehensive data collection and more on an internalized yet systemic understanding and discrimination of patients' symptoms and presentations. In his book *The Wisdom Paradox*,[2] Elkhonon Goldberg describes the changes he observed in himself as he approached 60: 'Previously, I dealt more with problem solving; nowadays I deal more with pattern recognition. I no longer have the expertise I used to for tiring, focused, work-intensive calculations ... More than once, when I face what seems to be a challenging problem, I somehow circumvent the tiresome step-by-step thought process ... The solution seems to arrive by itself, complete, without an effort.'[3]

Piaget's celebrated theory of the development of human thought assumes that our cognitive processes develop in childhood and reach a peak in adulthood, signalling the completion of the development of formal thinking. New studies have demonstrated that in our later years we develop a new way of thinking, known as postformal thought.[4] The transformation from 'formal thinking' to 'postformal thinking' is not a regression, but rather a necessary structural change. Our life experience teaches us that the answers to life's challenging questions cannot be classified as simply 'right' or 'wrong', as we most likely assumed while using formal thinking. As they age, a person gradually develops a relativist attitude to life issues, based on experience. It would be impossible to manage each challenge we face in life by separating them into independent variables and dealing with each one in isolation, as required by formal thinking. Rather, in the postformal thought phase of life, sensitivity to context becomes more important than detailed assumptions and general knowledge. As we gain years, we also gain the ability to make more intuitive decisions.

Intuition is often mistakenly viewed as a pre-analytical phenomenon. However, in his book *Thinking, Fast and Slow,* Nobel Prize winner Professor Daniel Kahneman begs to differ.[5] According to Kahneman, this kind of intuition of is a postformal ability based on the great store of wisdom which has accumulated in our richly developed 'mind maps'.[6] This postformal intelligence does not negate the importance of formal thinking, which at the same time keeps it in proportion. Those with well-developed postformal thinking do not surrender their ability to draw logical conclusions. However, they attribute more importance to what they've gained from their life experience, and to the implications of this, which they can apply to specific contexts. For younger people, their thought processes tend to be based on formal logic and its pre-determined problem-solving schema. However, as people age, their thinking transitions from logical sequencing to more open-ended, deeper thought processes.

Although it is likely that people gain the ability to use this open-ended thinking during their middle years, at the same time they often don't recognize, use or appreciate it. This may be because as adults, people are usually assessed by their formal thinking abilities. Following retirement, when people leave behind the structures which value formal thinking, the need and ability to activate postformal thinking skills become apparent.

As postformal thought skills are activated, they engender an enhanced sensitivity and wisdom. People can better identify the things that can be changed, make peace with those that can't be changed and gain the ability to distinguish between the two. Acceptance of what lies ahead makes it possible, both cognitively and emotionally, to start a new period of life, one characterized by interiority and a new knowledge of oneself and one's world. In other words, people's emotional intelligence is enhanced as they get older.

The head of a hospital department shared the following story with me. Due to a chronic personnel shortage, he had asked one of the retired nurses to come back to work, even on a part-time basis, simply to ease the unit's workload. She agreed and rejoined the team. Her boss found that since her retirement, her work style had undergone some qualitative changes. Her ability to cope with the tense interpersonal relationships of the department's overworked staff had improved, and she was a calming influence on her colleagues. He also found that her diagnostic abilities had vastly improved. She was outperforming not only the current staff, but her own pre-retirement self.

These abilities, which develop as we age, are precisely the ones necessary for creative activity. The commonly held belief that our creativity declines as we age is not supported by the evidence. There are many well-documented examples of creative people, such as artists and thinkers, who did not lose their creative abilities as they aged. Rather, creativity is enriched as it changes and develops.[7] The Italian Renaissance painter, Titian, created one of his most famous works at the age of 98; Goethe finished his dramatic masterpiece, *Faust*, at 83; the pianist Arthur Rubinstein was still playing with astonishing skill at 89. The ability to continue and develop our personal creativity is not limited to artists — rather, it exists in each one of us.

Creativity has many definitions. Common to all of them is the realization that our creative potential is dependent on a flexibility enabled by multi-dimensional, multi-directional thinking, which develops and improves as we age.[8] It is quite common to find that 'ordinary' people, who did not display any overt signs of creativity when young, discover it as they age. They start to draw or sculpt after they retire, uncovering their latent creativity.[9] In this context, it is important to note that creativity is not found only in areas like art, design, literature, music or philosophy.

Creativity has been defined as 'any new valuable solution to a problem within a given specific context'.[10] Even those who lacked the personal creativity to assure wise management of their lives during adulthood can acquire the necessary skills once retired.[11]

In sum, recent neurological and cognitive research indicates that we need to stop thinking of our later years as a period of inevitable decline, but rather regard them as an opportunity for personal growth and, indeed, for transforming the way in which we approach life.

Chapter 6

Creating New
'Mind Maps'

One of the most exciting recent discoveries in brain research is the extent to which the brain continues to be flexible at all ages. This flexibility is not lost even in advanced old age; it can persist and even grow stronger until we pass away.

To understand this discovery, we must first briefly explain how the brain works.

Every human brain has 100 billion nerve cells, called neurons. In addition, it has 30 billion synapses — electric and chemical transmitters linking the neurons. Each neuron has the potential for up to 30,000 such links. The brain can be viewed as an massive dynamic network which enables an almost endless number of such links. Potentially, each neuron can be connected to all the other neurons via these synapses.

As we focus attention on a particular issue or action, we activate our thoughts and emotions as well as our bodies. These trigger numerous pathways between different parts of the brain, creating dense networks of nerve cells and synapses which resemble trees. Brain scientists call the process by which these networks develop 'arborization' — a tree-like branching which makes new synaptic connections.

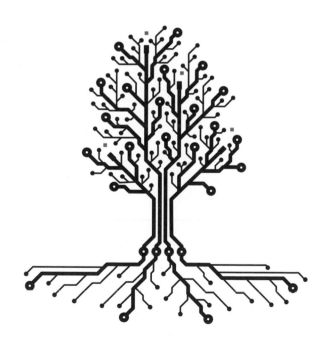

A STYLIZED REPRESENTATION OF ARBORIZATION

Cognitively, this process activates a synergy of our thoughts and emotions, working in conjunction with our physical and social functioning. The cognitive connections between words, ideas, emotions and actions can be represented as a 'mind map'.[1] The more we feel, think about and otherwise experience a particular issue and its various aspects, the more it enriches the relevant mind map we hold in our brain.

Like any other muscle in our body, the brain's elasticity requires training for its preservation. When you experience, feel, think and generally work it hard, its flexibility grows, and so its capacity and abilities improve.

The more you use your brain, the more efficient its neurons become, and fewer are needed to perform a specific action. Even the functioning of the synapses improves. Increased activity enables the transmission of information between the neurons to be more efficient.

A child who has just started to play the piano will tend to use their entire upper body — hand, arm and shoulder — to produce a single note. Even the mouth will contract with the effort. However, with practice, the child will learn to use a single finger to produce the required note, without exercising unnecessary muscles. Rather than the huge number of neurons conscripted to perform the original action, the well-practised brain needs only a handful of specialized cells which are perfectly suited for the task. These specialized neurons can process data very quickly, without investing much thought in performing the activity.

On the other hand, when we no longer challenge our brains, our mind maps weaken and atrophy. This is the double-edged sword of elasticity, or indeed of most skills: if you don't use it, you lose it.

One of the best-known studies of the brain's agility involved London taxi drivers. Some large cities, like New York or Paris, have a grid of avenues and streets which help drivers find their way around; however, in London navigation is a much more difficult task, as the streets do not follow an easily recognizable pattern. Training London's cabbies takes 2–4 years, during which time they must learn to recognize the 25,000 streets and thousands of public places in the city. Subsequently, the drivers undergo a series of memory tests and simulated navigation exercises which cover almost 100 kilometres (60 miles) of streets and include traffic signs, street lights and pedestrians, as well as cab and bus traffic.

The study, which used fMRI images of the drivers' brains, was carried out by Professor Elinor McGuire and her research group from the University of London.[2] It demonstrated that the arborization of London cabbies' brains, along with their mind maps, is far richer and more elastic than those of other drivers, like you and me, and even of London bus drivers. This is because, unlike bus drivers, cabbies are required to go to many different destinations according to customers' requests, to improvise and to find shortcuts. On the other hand, cabbies who had retired or changed jobs showed diminished levels of arborization, as well as deterioration of their driving mind maps.

To generalize: when we specialize in a particular field, our brain creates a mind map of that field, based on the skills we have acquired. So if you're a teacher, you have a teaching mind map; if you're a civil engineer, you have a civil engineering mind map; if you're a bank manager, you have a bank manager's mind map. However, when we retire, and cease the activities and actions which characterized our working life, the mind maps which had served us so well weaken and atrophy.

Therefore, to keep our brains active and agile after retirement, we need to develop new mind maps which suit the new circumstances of our life. To achieve this, we must activate our brains intensively and mindfully.

The more aware we are of our changing circumstances, and the more we invest in seeking new ways to solve the problems which they raise, the better equipped we will be to create and enrich new mind maps. The problem is that most of us are not aware of the need to do this, nor do we know how to do so mindfully.

In 2007, psychoanalyst Norman Doidge published *The Brain that Changes Itself*, where he discusses the amazing elasticity of the human brain and suggests that we view it as a dynamic, adaptable organ which can be consciously modified by its users.[3] Doidge's book has sold more than a million copies worldwide and has also stimulated a great deal of subsequent research and writing. Despite all this work, the influence of our mind maps on the aging process, and how they might reverse or at lease slow the brain's aging, have remained largely unexplored.

In the following chapters, I set out to remove some of the mystery surrounding how we can activate the brain's elasticity as we age. At this point, I would like simply to stress that these new findings on the brain's elasticity, even in our advanced years, enable us to define and understand old age in a new way.

Neurologically, wc bccomc old when our adult mind maps are no longer in use and we have not made the effort to create new mind maps that will enable us to cope with the changing conditions of our lives. I concur with British writer George Orwell, best known for his dystopian novel *Nineteen Eighty-four*. According to him, death does not begin when the heart stops. Rather, death starts when a person loses the ability to think of new ways of achieving self-fulfillment and becomes resigned to the repetition of the same old things, trapped by the same old thoughts.

Chapter 7

The Age of Wisdom: A New Phase of Life

I have suggested that people have the potential to enjoy a new and meaningful period of life between retirement and geriatric old age. Despite this prospect, we are still captured by the paradigm of three distinct phases of life: childhood, adulthood and old age.

The commonly held conception is that retirement marks the passage from adulthood to old age, despite the twenty-year increase in life expectancy following retirement. We do not ask ourselves whether it is natural for a human being to have twenty years of sabbatical.

We all need vacations. However, when they become too long, our peace of mind slowly evaporates. In the end, even holidays can become routine and boring;

we can end spending our time restlessly searching for anything to fill the void.

Summing up what I have learned so far on my journey of enquiry, I again pose the question: why should we assume that we 'officially' enter old age when we retire?

My findings have led me to conclude that the social and personal revolution inherent in the dramatic rise in life expectancy should not be viewed as a quantitatively prolonged downhill process, ending in death. Rather, it should be considered as a qualitative revolution in human life, a new period of life which provides us with new horizons we could not have imagined before. This period is inherently different from the adulthood which precedes it and the old age which follows it.

In previous centuries, there was no point in seeking to mindfully shape the post-retirement years as they were so few in number. It made sense to view any post-work years as a brief bonus at the end of life. However, now most of us have been granted twenty or more post-retirement years and the new opportunities this brings. In view of current knowledge in neurology and medicine, there is no reason for us not to fully enjoy this new period and delay 'old age' to the very end of life.

This can be a time which provides us with a chance to experience another round of active life — wiser, more meaningful and even more enjoyable than the life we had as adults. In adulthood we are often overburdened with managing our careers, combined with the demands of building families and raising children.

The post-retirement period gives us a new freedom to design and experience more fulfilling and balanced lives.

I call this new period of life 'the age of wisdom'. The name exemplifies its essential quality. In coining the name, I have followed the Jewish scriptures, which differentiate between 'cleverness' and 'wisdom'. In the book of *Proverbs*, chapter 3, verse 13, King Solomon writes: 'A clever person is one who knows how to learn from others. A wise person is one who knows how to go beyond what he has learned from others.' In other words, wisdom is a quality that is extrapolated from one's own experience and awareness.

According to Benjamin Franklin, 'Life's tragedy is that we get old too soon and wise too late.' This was indeed the case until recently. However, with the extension of life a long way past retirement age, we now have the time to apply our hard-earned wisdom to enjoy this new period of our lives.

Apparently, we are the only species which cannot escape awareness of our own lives, as well our inevitable end. In youth and adulthood, we are preoccupied with life and living while ignoring our inevitable end. On the other hand, in our later years, when we are all too aware of our impending death, reframing our future seems pointless. However, the rise in life expectancy has created a new phase of human existence, one where the consciousness of life and death meet. This in turn enables us to use the wisdom we have gained to ponder our lives and change direction, so that we can maximize the extra years we have been granted.

The wisdom phase of our life offers us new opportunities to make qualitative changes to our lives so as to enhance not only our personal experience, but our surroundings and society at large.

Unlike old age, this is a period of personal growth rather than decline — despite the health problems we face, and the difficulties and losses which are inevitable as we get older. It opens a new, wider perspective on human life.

The identification of a new stage in human life, and the resultant opportunities for shaping our lives, goes against the deeply entrenched belief that life is comprised of three periods: childhood, adulthood and old age.

However, the rejection of this traditional triadic division becomes easier to accept when we understand that youth, as a distinct and separate stage of life between childhood and adulthood, was only recognized less than 200 years ago. Before that, in traditional societies, childhood ended at age thirteen, when boys joined the adult hunters and when puberty made girls eligible for motherhood. In Judaism, at thirteen a boy becomes responsible for keeping the edicts of Jewish law and is considered an adult. Adulthood was the longest phase of people's lives, lasting from about the age of ten to 40 or 45. It was followed by a short 'old age', ending in what we would now consider premature death.

At the beginning of the Industrial Revolution, child labour was commonplace. The transition from childhood to adulthood occurred earlier, as children eight to ten years old found themselves in production and assembly lines. However, as the Industrial Revolution matured, longer training periods were required for professions like engineering and accounting. This in turn triggered an opposite trend — delayed entry to the workforce.

In tandem with new laws prohibiting child employment, the need for lengthier training and education gave rise to a new phase of life between childhood and adulthood — youth. Now, at the beginning of the 21st century, we are witnessing the evolution of another new period in the human journey from life to death — the age of wisdom.

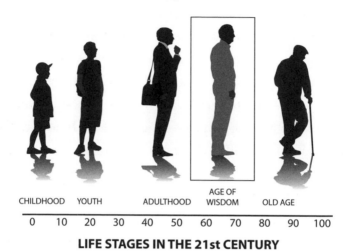

LIFE STAGES IN THE 21st CENTURY

Illustration © Zvi Lanir

At the moment, very few people know how to take advantage of this new stage. There is almost no public awareness of the implications of the wisdom period for society and the economy. Such understanding will take time. This was also the case with youth: Only gradually did it become recognized as a separate stage in human life with its own characteristics, needs and implications.

During the nineteenth century and the beginning of the twentieth, youth become a subject of academic study and research as a separate entity. This research highlighted the importance of this stage to human development and well-being, as well as to society and the economy.

Contemporary society recognizes the many benefits which the life-stage of youth has contributed to our development as individuals and as a society. Its function as a catalyst for social and economic development is unique. Nowadays, the 'age of youth' plays a major part in the entrepreneurial risk-taking and technological innovation undertaken by startup companies.

The process which led to the recognition of 'the age of youth' as a separate stage of human life took many years. We can only hope that the social recognition of the age of wisdom will be accomplished more rapidly, as contemporary society is characterized by a higher level of self-awareness and advanced networking tools for the dissemination of new ideas.

In any case, it makes no sense for us as individuals to continue to accept the social norm which views retirement as the beginning of old age, thereby imprisoning ourselves within a self-fulfilling prophecy.

Chapter 8

The First Hurdle: Ageism

We tend to classify anyone who is retired as 'old', even when thinking about ourselves. Moving beyond this socially imposed stigma is a big challenge. In fact, this is the first hurdle which we must overcome in order to recognize and experience the wisdom period of our lives.

The reasons for accepting this classification are complex. Broadly speaking, society defines anyone who has retired as 'old'. This definition relates only to an individual's chronological age, ignoring their functional age. This universally accepted attitude is the root cause of ageism.

The term 'ageism' was coined by Robert Butler — MD, psychologist and gerontologist — to denote age-based discrimination.[1] The word reminds us of other well-known discriminatory practices: racism, discrimination based on race, and sexism, discrimination based on gender.

Like racism and sexism, ageism is prevalent in the workplace. It is based on a nexus of stereotypes. Older people have supposedly lost the ability to handle change, are unable to acquire new skills and are less efficient and productive.

By contrast, the labour market actively seeks out people in their twenties; those in the 45–50 age group struggle to find new jobs. Nobody wants to hire workers whose best years seem to be behind them when young people in their prime can be hired, kept on staff for many years and require lower starting salaries.

Almost all countries have national retirement laws. These usually allow employers to release workers when they reach a pre-defined retirement age, with no compulsion to consider their actual functional abilities.

However, ageism is evident far beyond the workplace, in both the personal and the social spheres of life. External signs of aging like white hair and wrinkles trigger negative stereotypical reactions. These stereotypes include the perception of an older person as someone who walks and thinks slowly, whose interests, activities and curiosity are severely limited.

According to this way of thinking, the elderly are closed to the world, live in the past and have no real future, while their minds and bodies are shrinking in tandem.

Conventional expectations about old age are contrary. On the one hand, the elderly are urged to make efforts to slow down the decline towards geriatric old age. At the same time, they are told that they should use their 'golden years' to enjoy what capacities they have left.

When we retire, we become objects of the burgeoning 'old age' market, whose business is predicated on our fears of aging. Among other things, this market offers pharmacological products, food additives, anti-aging medication and plastic surgery companies and services.

Many entities claim to be experts in taking care of us once we've reached old age. These include public as well as private health-care organizations, rest homes and insurance companies. All of them try to convince us that a longer life expectancy is dependent on greater use of their services.

Social, institutional and commercial norms all work to reinforce our internal, built-in ageism, which is the hardest to rid ourselves of. Sigmund Freud explained why it is so difficult for us to discard our most cherished beliefs. According to Freud, internalization is a supremely important mechanism for successful socialization from the time we come into the world. It continues to guide our perceptions and behaviour throughout our lives. Using this mechanism, we internalize images, behavioural norms and social taboos. We also make them a part of us and turn them into the system of mental imagery which drives our perceptions of ourselves.

The internalization of the need to fit our behaviour to social expectations continues to shape our perceptions and expectations about ourselves when we retire.

The United Nations has recognized ageism as another form of discrimination, just like racism and sexism. Nevertheless, the battle against ageism has not yet taken off, as it has not received the level of attention given to racism and sexism. The main reason for this neglect seems to be a lack of awareness and organization by seniors themselves.

Mass protests have been pivotal in publicizing racism and sexism, educating both the general population and governments about the injustices involved. The conditions which have mobilized whole communities so against these forms of discrimination do not yet exist for ageism. Public awareness can only flow from personal awareness. Unfortunately, most of us are still not prepared to overturn our own ageism bias, even though all of us will suffer from it sooner or later.

To combat our internal ageism, we must first create a safe space for this newly acknowledged period in our lives and legitimize it for ourselves. Unfortunately, we still don't have the vocabulary necessary to interpret the meaning of retirement, other than the conventional terms used to describe old age. These commonly used terms for old age and its attendant features determine our beliefs, whether consciously or unconsciously, and imprison us within a self-defined cage of ageism.

The very concept of 'retirement' is misleading, as it suggests that life after work is an inevitable downhill road, ending in death.

A retired person usually receives a pension. This sends the message that while compensation is required for work done in the past, any further contribution to society is no longer expected.

Retirees are viewed as having left life's active playing field and are expected to negotiate the pitfalls of old age as best and as comfortably as they can. At the same time, it is expected that pensions will become increasingly inadequate as life's needs eat into their accumulated savings.

This anticipated decline is not limited to financial concerns. It includes the knowledge, wisdom and respect acquired during adulthood. With these, too, we start to gnaw away at the accumulated balance of our 'earnings' to date.

Society has devised a number of terms which give a positive veneer to people's lives after they have retired, such as 'senior citizen' and the 'golden years'. However, such expressions are little more than a comforting deception — a way of reclassifying people who have retired as 'old', while hinting that they have not yet gone 'over the hill' into geriatric old age.

Phrases such as 'You don't really look old' or 'You look younger than your years' are commonly used to describe people whose behaviour and looks do not fit with their chronological 'old' age. Many people have called me a 'young old person'. Lacking a new vocabulary, people cling to the old one and end up using a combination of familiar terms — 'young' and 'old'.

We all take a measure of comfort in repeating the truism that we get older a lot slower than we used to. 'Today's 70 is the new 50' is a familiar platitude. Many of my contemporaries claim that they are not as old as their chronological age. Nevertheless, we continue to view ourselves within the framework of old age as we know it. The familiar set of terms we all use to describe old age makes it hard for us to conceptualize ourselves outside this box.

Finding a New Vocabulary

In a nutshell, the struggle against our own internal ageism is also a battle against the language and terms we have grown up with. The words available to us are based on what we think we know about old age and reflect the popular imagery and needs associated with it. However, at the start of the 21st century, what we are experiencing about aging reflects a new and different kind of reality, one which we have not yet learned to express.

When I lecture about the 'hidden age', most of my audience react in the same way: 'We have a sense of this hidden age, but lack the words to name our feelings. What you've done is give us new words with which to process our feelings about this phase of our lives. This has helped us put these feelings and thoughts in perspective.'

I've been asked many times why I insist on talking about 'the age of wisdom' or 'the wisdom years' rather than 'young old age'. Why shouldn't we retain the term 'old age' to describe this stage of life? For example,

Jewish tradition views old age as the peak of intelligence and spirituality, rather than as the beginning of one's inevitable decline towards death. It views old people as role models for society and as conduits of wisdom and knowledge for subsequent generations.

However, this idyllic image is not supported by the way in which old people have been seen in most societies. During most of human history, old age has usually been quite short. It was commonly viewed as a pointless appendage to human life, following the completion of the task of bringing the next generation into the world and providing for it. Old age heralded the change from a person's status as an asset to an economic and social liability. Of course, this outlook influenced society's attitude to old people, both consciously and subconsciously. The prevalent image of the 'elders' of a community who gain respect through their knowledge and experience is just that — an image unsupported by the facts. While most religions pay lip service to the need to honour one's parents, in reality old people were commonly marginalized and banished to a life of loneliness and poverty.

The current attitude to old age dictates what is expected of us once we retire. It defines what is right for us and what is not, how we should dress, move and even feel. It sets up a restrictive belief system within which we are expected to function, thus structuring our everyday reality.

For these reasons, I have consistently opposed any attempt to include the word 'old' in any description of this new period in our lives. I continue to insist on the title of 'the age of wisdom'. By using the word 'wisdom', I am offering a nucleus around which a new set of concepts — and a new vocabulary — for our thoughts and actions in later life can crystallize.

The creation of a new mindset involves a long and complicated sociological process. It leaves people like me, who are part of the first generation to experience this new life stage, feeling stranded. Previous generations took exclusion from the field of active life, and relegation to old age, somewhat for granted. Now we feel that we are in a double bind. On the one hand, we are unwilling to take this negative attitude 'sitting down', as we know that our abilities, feelings and desires have taken some giant steps forward. On the other hand, perception, language and knowledge have not kept pace with these changes, leaving us in a kind of limbo.

As a result, we find ourselves in uncharted conceptual territory, without roads and footpaths, without landmarks and without lights to mark our way. Up till now, we kept to the paths which society had carefully and clearly marked out for us — childhood, youth, adulthood and old age. Our parents knew that our paths must lead us through child care and school. As teenagers we had to finish high school with a diploma, followed by some tertiary training, whether academic or vocational. Society further marked out our way by pressuring us to choose a career, train for it and then develop it over our time in the workforce. Getting married and building a family, acquiring a home and a mortgage, going back to school for further training, climbing the corporate ladder — all these steps were clearly and explicitly expected of us along the path of life.

However, once we retire, these familiar road signs disappear and there are no new goals and no new summits to scale. We are simply expected to accept becoming old. If we acquiesce, society will provide us with clear guidelines about how to act and what to expect in our remaining years. Unlike the active instructions that marked out our path during youth and adulthood, these are passive directives.

However, if we want to experience the post-retirement years as a new life stage, different from 'old age', we don't yet know how to proceed. Society has not yet formulated guidelines for realizing the potential of this new period of our lives.

Only when my journey had brought me to this point did I understood that I am in effect an explorer in uncharted territory, attempting to mark out new paths in a conceptual desert — not just for myself, but for others as well.

In Parts Two and Three, I will attempt to set up a few beacons to light the path ahead.

PART TWO

Towards a Theory of the
Wisdom Years

Chapter 9

Understanding the Psychological Foundations of the Wisdom Years

The search for a theoretical foundation that would allow us to understand the processes we need to undergo in order to experience the wisdom years led me to the next stage of my journey of discovery — the realm of developmental psychology. What do developmental psychologists have to say about human development in the later years?

Every discussion of developmental psychology begins with Sigmund Freud. Freud was the first to propose a theory that describes how the human personality is formed. However, Freud focused on the formation of personality in childhood, and did not consider the possibility of new personality development in the later stages of life.

Concerning himself with human development from the point of view of childhood, Freud regarded adulthood as the stage of life in which a person completes the process of psychological formation, thus allowing individuals to fulfill the two major roles associated with adulthood — work and love. When a person withdraws from love and work, they withdraw from life — all that lies beyond the period of love and work is old age, in which no further personality development is to be expected.

Carl Jung, Freud's famous student, was in his 30s when Freud appointed him as his professional heir. But only a few years later the two psychoanalysts parted ways and became rivals. The background to their split was, among other things, Jung's disagreement with Freud's focus on childhood development as the key to human personality. Jung believed that attention should be paid to a person's development on a continuing basis — including after they have resolved the conflicts of childhood and fulfilled the demands of family and work.

In Jung's view, after a person has completed the period of active adulthood, with its particular duties and responsibilities, they can — and must — allow themselves to pay attention to their inner life, to understand themselves more deeply and thus to reframe their identity.

Jung linked this ongoing inner development to the consciousness of approaching death — only when a person is willing to recognize their inevitable end have they sufficiently matured so as to establish a new and steadfast grip on life. People have an obligation to focus their attention and energy on the things that make life worthwhile. In Jung's view, this new focus on one's individual needs will lead to a renewed period of personal growth, enabling people to take full advantage of what life can offer in the later years.

To achieve these goals, one must undergo a process of personal transformation which Jung named 'individuation'. Individuation is the process by which a person becomes aware of the various interior aspects of their make-up and integrates them into a new functional entity.

During adulthood, we are subjected to social pressure to be similar to other people and to conform to social norms. When people finally allow themselves to be freed from these pressures, a new impulse emerges — the desire to understand and live one's life as a unique individual.

This inward convergence does not lead to egoism. On the contrary, through the process of individuation, each person becomes more socially conscious and more willing to contribute to the well-being of others and to society and humanity as whole — or, as Jung puts it: 'Individuation does not sever a person from the world, but helps him to gather the world into himself.'

The stage of life which I have dubbed 'the age of wisdom' was described by Jung as 'the second adulthood period'. He emphasized that if, during this period, the potential for personal growth is not realized, the negative symptoms of old age will inevitably manifest themselves — dogmatism, defensiveness, an obsessive preoccupation with the past, boredom, suffering and depression.[1]

In the 1950s, the psychologist Erik Erikson developed the influential 'stages of psychosocial development' theory that divides human life into eight stages. The seventh stage is 'midlife adulthood', which he characterized — probably influenced by Jung's views — as the period in which a person engages in a personal struggle to find meaning in life.

Erikson distinguishes between midlife adulthood and the last stage of human life — 'old age'. Like Jung, Erikson argued that in the first half of their adult life people are too busy to ask questions about the meaning and purpose of life, but after completing what society sees as the duties of adulthood, 'more parts of the person himself want to emerge; now he is ready to raise questions about the meaning of all this to him and his happiness.'

According to Erikson, asking these questions may lead to what he described as 'the midlife crisis', later better known as the '40-year-old crisis'. However, studies conducted since the 1980s indicate that most of us do not experience the phenomenon that Erikson described as the midlife crisis in our 40s. A recent research study found that whereas in 1978, 80 per cent of respondents said that they had experienced such a crisis at the age of 40, in a similar poll conducted in 1985, only 70 per cent claimed to have experienced the 40-year-old crisis, and in recent years less than 10 per cent of Americans have reported experiencing a significant psychological crisis in their 40s.[2]

What happened? Where did the 40-year-old crisis go? It did not disappear. With the increase in life expectancy, it has probably just been postponed, to appear in a more acute form ten or twenty years later. The increase in life expectancy has displaced the 40-year-old crisis, transformed it and made it more severe.

Whenever it actually strikes, this crisis is conventionally related to the so-called menopausal changes in women, which mark the end of the period of fertility and the beginning of physical decline. In men, this period is characterized by decreased libido and erectile quality. In both women and men, there is a reduction in muscular mass, the onset of osteoporosis, increased body fat, degenerative changes in the skin and hair loss.

All these changes occur in parallel to the 'empty nest' phenomenon. It becomes more severe when it coincides with retirement and the feeling that 'the children no longer need us'. On top of all this, the consciousness of one's approaching death becomes ever more tangible.

The crisis sparked by these changes brings the individual to a critical life crossroads that Erikson describes as 'integrity versus despair'. The successful negotiation of this crisis creates a new sense of personal integrity and self-worth. However, failure to deal with this crisis drags a person down to a place of despair, bitterness and a fearful consciousness of personal mortality.

The Individuation Process

Following Jung and Erikson, more recent researchers in human development have applied the concept of individuation to define the parameters of personality development in two earlier stages of life. The first is the process of separation — individuation of the infant from the mother. This stage has been described by the psychologist Margaret Mahler as the process of shaping the infant as an independent, separate personality.[3] This stage normally lasts until the age of three, when the baby completes its separation from the mother and develops an ego and a distinct identity of its own. The success of this separation or individuation process is a key factor in determining the child's future development.

The second individuation in human life was identified by the psychopathologist Peter Blos as taking place during adolescence and early adulthood.[4] What in infancy is 'a hatching from the symbiotic membrane to become an individual toddler' is mirrored, during adolescence, by a separation from family dependency and a transition to an identification with the individual's own age group as he or she gradually becomes a member of the adult world. Failure to negotiate this second period of individuation may be expressed in an absence of purpose, chronic procrastination and extreme mood swings.

The third manifestation of individuation — one that is intended to usher the individual into the wisdom years — is substantially different from the two earlier phases. In both of these, society and culture are major actors in the process, providing established guidelines for negotiating them. When the process is successful, the person concerned is seen as slipping seamlessly into their new role.

The third and final individuation process is very different. Here, the individual finds themself alone. Because society is unaware of the need to undertake such a process, those making the transition find themselves facing it without any guidance on how to proceed.

While in the first two individuation processes individuals have no need to consciously orient themselves to a particular procedure or role, in the third transition, the person must learn how to proceed in a conscious, individual manner — in many cases contrary to the powerful messages conveyed by society.

While the individuation of adolescence was mainly oriented to becoming a full member of society, those making this third transition must prepare themselves for an interior withdrawal. Now, the individual is required to reconnect with themselves, to contemplate their inner self, to learn to recognize it and to connect with the parts of the personality that have been suppressed until now, to experience them as legitimate components of the whole and to recruit

all of them to face the increasing hardships of aging —
all without missing out on the advantages presented by
the wisdom years.

Jung claimed that this process of individuation
has a holistic healing effect, both mentally and
physically, enabling the individual to delay and cope
more effectively with the hardships of old age.

The psychosocial individuation discussed above is
a creative process involving the emotional, cognitive
and functional faculties that, if navigated successfully,
enables new growth in a person's self-perception and
functioning. It entails dealing with questions — new
and old — about one's self and one's attitude towards
self and the world. This process does not involve
abstract philosophical and psychological questions,
but rather is related to a person's motivation to create
a deep and spontaneous connection with both their
inner and outer reality, and to find ways to circumvent
the difficulties that will inevitably be encountered in a
holistic way.

For Jung, and to a large extent Erikson as well,
the process of individuation was seen as a psychiatric
treatment issue. However, the approach adopted in
this book is different. My aim is to offer readers the
knowledge, the encouragement and the ability to cope
with the processes involved, on their own account.

Thus we need a theory that is not just based in psychology, but is essentially cognitive in nature, one that will answer the question: what are the skills and procedures needed to successfully complete such a process? These will be the subject of chapters 10 and 11.

Chapter 10

How Our Brains Work: The Challenges Ahead

In order to understand how individuals can consciously influence their cognitive processes to make the personal changes they need in later life, we need to know how our brain works.

Most of the brain (about 80 per cent by weight and volume) is contained in the cerebral cortex. This ball-like mass is divided by a deep groove into two main hemispheres — the right and left hemispheres. At the base of the brain is the posterior lobe, known as the primal brain.

Although these three brain lobes have developed on different evolutionary time scales, they function in an integrated manner. While the way that each of these lobes function is remarkable in itself, even more remarkable is how they work together.

The Primal Brain

The primal brain is also called the reptilian brain, because it is the main brain found in reptiles. Its development in humans occurred long before the development of the frontal lobes and human development as an intelligent creature.

It is also the first brain that develops in newborns. The infant emerges into the world equipped with a brain which enables them to activate breathing, control the heartbeat and carry out sucking, excretion and other functions essential to life.

The primal brain is our least-valued brain. We are insufficiently aware of its sophistication and its comprehensive impact on us. It enables all our motor and physical functions, actions which we perform automatically.

These functions served our primeval ancestors well in situations where it was necessary to co-ordinate vital body systems to ensure concentrated, co-ordinated and rapid action — the 'fight or flight' response. To survive, ancient humans had to focus on the many dangers around them and ignore anything that would distract them from the keys tasks of avoiding predation and success in hunting. Our primal brain was designed to perform these functions automatically.

It is thanks to the primal brain that we can recognize a face in a crowd instinctively, even before we consciously activate our thinking processes. Studies monitoring subjects' responses using fMRI scans have demonstrated that when shown images on a computer screen, they reacted by pressing a particular key while still debating what to choose with the 'conscious' part of the brain. In these experiments, the subjects acted before they were aware of what they were doing.

Today, while we are rarely involved in fight-or-flight situations, these functions are activated when someone irritates or threatens us. Our pulse quickens, our breath shortens, we start sweating and we react almost without self-control.

Many of our reactive characteristics derive from the basic need to survive in a hostile world, situations which our ancestors routinely faced millions of years ago. This is the reason for our tendency to think in set patterns and to judge according to strongly rooted templates, even when we have only very partial information about a situation.

The mind of the animal fighting for survival is focused on scanning for potential threats — where will the predator come from? Today we no longer need to employ such constant vigilance, but nevertheless our minds are continually overwhelmed by worries and fears.

Our brain, when not focused on the reflective thinking that requires the activation of our frontal lobes, occupies itself, obsessively, in passing from fear to fear and from worry to worry — without helping us find solutions to this free-floating anxiety stream. Did I lock the door before I left the house? Will the meeting finish in time for me to pick up my son from school? What will happen if my overdraft keeps on growing?

When we retire, we become especially vulnerable to this aspect of the reptile brain. The mental vacuum created by retirement may be filled with disturbing thoughts and worries. It is at this critical time in our lives that we need to focus on filling this vacuum with new sensations and thoughts by consciously activating the two frontal hemispheres of the brain.

The Right Hemisphere

The right hemisphere is responsible for emotion, imagination and creativity. Like the posterior lobe, the right hemisphere of the brain is not unique to humans. Other mammals also have it but, having succeeded in modifying the function of the right hemisphere, humans have expanded their world far beyond what other mammals are capable of.

Until about 60,000 years ago, the range of thought, emotion and imagination possessed by humans was, like other mammals, limited to what could be perceived by the senses. Like other animals, early humans could communicate in sign language and warn one another of an approaching predator. They could also envisage various scenarios, solve problems and develop tools, but these were limited to their sensory range. Our ability to feel and imagine things that exist beyond the range of the senses began to develop gradually, comparatively recently in evolutionary terms.

It was this development in the brain that gradually enabled humans to think not only about things restricted to the realm of the senses, but also to consider things that did not exist in the reality of their quotidian world — to imagine, and to create new realities.

These new abilities gradually enabled the development of art, poetry, religion and democracy, the invention of money and the monetary system, and the establishment of corporations and the stock market. All these cultural forms and institutions could never have come into being without the ability of humans to imagine and describe things that do not yet exist in reality.[1] It is precisely this capacity that has enabled me to develop the concept of a new stage of life — the age of wisdom.

To successfully implement the individuation process required by the wisdom years, we will need to consciously activate the skill set associated with the right hemisphere of our brains — which will in turn enable us to sense the changes we are undergoing, to imagine the new possibilities before us, and to direct our thinking, actions and behaviour to overcome — or at least manage — the crises that await us all in later life.

In sum, the right hemisphere will play an important role enabling us to reimagine, reinterpret and reactualize ourselves.

The Left Hemisphere

The left hemisphere, which is responsible for our linguistic and logical abilities, is likewise not unique to humans and can be found in other mammals — which also enjoy some linguistic and logical abilities.

It is difficult to know when ancient humans developed the linguistic and logical thinking skills that distinguish them. Most commentators believe that it happened around 30,000 years ago. The first known written language dates from around 5000 years ago.

The imaginative faculty, which had already developed in the right hemisphere, was the foundation on which our linguistic and logical capacities, acquired mainly by the left hemisphere, could be developed.

Finally, the combined power of the two hemispheres made possible the development of science around 3000 years ago.

During the first two years of a baby's life, the right hemisphere of the brain develops rapidly. The right hemisphere controls our brains for the first three years of our lives. Only then does the left hemisphere begin to grow.

Twenty-six-month-old infants are right-brain creatures who experience and conceptualize themselves and their surroundings through emotion and imagination, but can hardly speak about what they are feeling and imagining.

In the first two years of life, the mother mainly communicates with her baby nonverbally, activating the brain's right hemisphere to 'reach' the baby's right brain. In order for an infant to become familiar with and control their emotions, and make social connections, he or she must experience this reciprocity hundreds of times during this critical period, and also receive the kind of encouragement that will reinforce these connections.

The child's move from preschool to primary school largely marks the transition from the dominance of the right brain to control by the left brain. When we enter adulthood, in order to climb the career ladder and advance professionally, we rely to a great extent on the left hemisphere of our brains.

As adults, we tend to attribute supreme importance to our logical skills; as far as we are concerned, this is the main function of the brain. We are taught to identify sound thinking with logic, and to treat our feelings and emotions as inferior because they are 'not logical'. The conventional assumption is that our feelings mislead us and, in order to act rationally, we need to control our emotions. This despite the fact that intuition and imagination play an important role in any scientific discovery, which we mistakenly assume is driven by pure logic.

Combining the Functions of our Three Lobes

The connection between the right and left hemispheres is achieved by the corpus callosum, which allows us to transfer what we feel and imagine in the right lobe to the logical judgment of the left hemisphere. Their synergetic relationship plays an important role in all human progress.

Although we are unaware of it, we cannot describe our world and even our daily lives without concepts that were initially imagined and then transformed into reality through logical processes. Thus, for example, the measurement we call a metre does not exist in nature — after being conceived in the right hemisphere, the concept then was processed logically by the left hemisphere of our brains. The thought processes that led to the invention of the wheel, car and plane, as well as the computer, the internet and social networks all took the same course.

The synergetic relationship between the right and left hemispheres plays an important role in our personal development as well. This capability of our brain is what enables us to think about, and initiate, fundamental changes in our personal lives — changes which go beyond the beliefs, behaviour and habits which society implants in us.

In order to rid ourselves of the once useful habits we acquired in adulthood, but which have now ceased to serve us, and indeed may even harm us, and to adopt new ones that are more compatible with the needs of the wisdom years, we must synergistically activate all three lobes of our brain. Not only the frontal right and left hemispheres, but also the lobe in charge of our automatic functions — the posterior lobe or primal brain, which plays an important role in acquiring new habits.

When we practise some activity, repeatedly performing a new action which simultaneously activates the three lobes of our brains, we can transform what we are performing into a newly learned habit — one which we will activate intuitively, without having to invest much thought in it.

The art of car parking offers a good example of this process. Our brains learn and get to know — intuitively — if the space between two parked cars will accommodate our vehicle, without us needing to make complex calculations of size and space, which would be time-consuming and likely not produce a better outcome.[2] The simultaneous activation of our three lobes enables us, following repeated practice, to gradually improve our ability to perform this everyday action rapidly and efficiently, and without the mental load that encumbered our initial attempts.

In order to achieve the individuation appropriate to the wisdom years, we will need to learn how to *consciously* activate the integration of the three lobes of our brains — this is not only a matter of changing perceptions, but also a question of changing habits,[3] and as such requires the collaboration of all three lobes.

Unlike the earlier phases of our lives, when we thought, felt and acted without thinking about the brain mechanisms engaged, because our mind maps were largely provided externally, we now find ourselves having to reorganize our whole way of life, purposefully and consciously exchanging our old mind maps for new ones.

So, when we retire, not only should we not allow our brains to retire, but we should also be aware that only by attaining a new level of awareness based on intensive activation of the brain can we reap the full benefits of the new life stage that lies before us.

Chapter 11

Renewing Mind and Body in Later Life

In recent years, neuroscientists have begun to uncover the circular connection between neurology and cognition. Our brains affect our thinking, but our thinking also changes our minds. Through active and conscious thinking during the wisdom years, we can positively influence the functioning of our brains.

The discovery of a feedback loop between cognition[1] and neurology surprised brain researchers, and caused them considerable embarrassment, as such a link flew in the face of established theories. Even today, many still find it difficult to accept the existence of a mechanism that connects neurology and cognition.

One of the first studies in which this circuit was detected was the so-called Nun Study, as it was carried out on a group of 678 Catholic nuns, members of the School Sisters of Notre Dame at their house near Mankato, Minnesota.[2] Beginning in 1986, the study was conducted by a team of researchers, headed by Professor David Snowdon of the University of Kentucky, who were interested in the development of Alzheimer's disease at advanced ages.

Nuns are a very convenient subject for scientific research because of their stable and uniform lifestyle. They do not smoke and do not drink much alcohol. They do not experience the physical changes associated with pregnancy, and they all eat the same foods. Most of the nuns in the study were engaged in the same occupation — as teachers in the school attached to their convent.

This group particularly interested the researchers because, statistically, nuns live longer than the general population. Indeed, most of the School Sisters lived for more than 90 years and among those participating in the study there were even a few centenarians.

Over a period of around fifteen years, the nuns were given numerous tests that examined various aspects of their cognitive functioning. They also agreed to donate their brains to the study after death, and thus it was possible to conduct a comparative study — to examine their cognitive function in old age and compare it to the neurological state of their brains after death.

The findings stunned the researchers — when they compared the post-mortem neurological evidence with cognitive follow-up data on their functioning as elderly women, it became clear that, in many of the subjects, there was a large gap between the two. Although signs of advanced Alzheimer's disease were found in the brains of some subjects, in life they showed no signs of mental decline. Most had continued to be alert and full of life, and had functioned well until shortly before their deaths.

In the wake of the Nun Study, other studies have also found discrepancies between neurological evidence of Alzheimer's disease, dementia and other neurodegenerative brain diseases, on the one hand, and the actual functioning of the people involved, on the other.[3]

Neurologists have given a name to this paradox: cognitive reserve.[4] A person who maintains an active lifestyle, continuing to cultivate their cognitive abilities throughout their lifespan, builds up a 'reserve' that enables them to continue functioning normally even when they are affected by degenerative diseases that attack the brain.[5]

The effects of cognitive reserve can be illuminated by an analogy from the computer world — our neurological condition can be compared to hardware, and cognition to software. Up to a certain level, updated software allows us to continue to perform the functions we require, even on a computer whose hardware performance is suboptimal. The software compensates for the 'degenerative aging' of the hardware.

Parallel to the discovery of cognitive reserve, neurobiology experienced another major shock after researchers discovered that the brains of adult mammals could produce new neurons. Previously, brain biologists had believed that the ability to produce new neurons was restricted to the young. However, in the early 1980s, a series of studies by Professor Elizabeth Gould of Rockefeller University found that new cells could also form in the brains of adult mice.

While Elizabeth Gould's studies were done on mice, in 1998 a Swedish–American team, led by Peter Eriksson of the Sahlgrenska University Hospital, Sweden, published a study in the academic journal *Nature Medicine* that demonstrated for the first time that the creation of new brain cells in a mature brain — neurogenesis — could also occur in the human adult brain.

These processes occur in the area of the brain called the hippocampus. This organ regulates a variety of brain functions including memory, learning, spatial orientation, mood and the emotions.

An adult can produce around 700 new cells a day. This might sound like a negligible number in a brain that has a hundred billion cells, but because the rate of death of brain cells increases as we age, this neurogenesis process may be of particular importance for the elderly.

The problem with these new brain cells is that they are not necessarily permanent. Many of them — even most of them — disappear a few weeks after they are formed. The short lifespan of these cells has prompted researchers to question why the brain produces new cells only to let them die off so rapidly.

The answer seems to be that the brain produces these cells 'just in case' they might be used. If a person is responding to the challenges life presents and using their brain actively and intensively, the cells remain. But if this is not the case, they disappear.

It is only dealing with new tasks that require considerable thought, and involve the brain in expending a continuous effort involving many brain cells, that prevents the new cells forming in elderly brains from dying.

In light of these findings, researchers distinguish two types of reserve — cognitive reserve and 'brain reserve'.

While cognitive reserve refers to the fact that humans exhibit a wide range of ability to function in regard to the aging processes of the brain, brain reserve refers to biological differences occurring within the brain itself.

Decay and Regeneration

Our ability to enhance our health, even at an advanced age, through physical activity and appropriate nutrition, to slow the deterioration of the body and create 'body reserve', has long been known. Brain research is showing that biological improvements in the brain are possible as well, even at an advanced age. This closes the circle. Through the choices we make, we can influence our personal aging process.

Aging is a natural process that we all experience throughout our lives. Developmental processes and aging processes are intertwined. In our bodies, growth and development occurs both through the expansion of the dimensions of existing cells and through the formation of new cells through division. However, there are limits to the number of times that a cell can be divided.

In childhood and adolescence, cell division primarily serves growth. In adulthood, the emphasis is shifted to preserving existing functions and repairing damage. Later, as the aging process progresses, the efficiency of our organs and tissues decreases. Cells lose their uniformity, their tissue arrangement becomes more random, their ability to metabolize decreases, the system that produces antibodies in the body becomes compromised and autoimmune diseases appear. Our body's ability to protect us from various threats decreases.

Our body is a very complex and sophisticated system. Like any system — no matter how complex and sophisticated it may be — it will ultimately wear out and die. Imagine a complex structure such as a power plant or a nuclear reactor. Safety engineers can tell us how such systems 'age' and then 'die'. They are designed to function for a long time without problems. However, while they have multiple backup systems, maintenance repairs are made from time to time and defective parts are replaced, the damage caused by wear and tear accumulates. The whole system deteriorates gradually, until eventually some minor random failure causes it to fail.

As human beings, we resemble these complex mechanical systems in various ways. We also have 'backups', which operate at all levels — from the cells, through the tissues and organs, to a whole system level. We are also subject to medical maintenance repairs, and even part replacements. What specialist maintenance engineers know as 'the degradation of complex systems' also applies to us. Like mechanical systems, in biological systems defects multiply over time and the system becomes weaker. Then the moment comes when a small unanticipated malfunction causes its collapse. Eventually, pneumonia, or one more seriously damaged artery, will carry us off. We wear out until we can wear out no longer.

Death occurs when the individual's ability to cope with this wear and tear no longer allows them to overcome the diseases and disorders that are always poised to attack. Then, minor problems — even a simple cold — can be fatal. When this happens, deterioration is very rapid and death can also come unexpectedly — within a few months, weeks, days or even hours.

The death certificate of someone who has died in old age will always list the final cause of death — respiratory insufficiency, cardiac arrest and so on. However, in such cases no single disease is responsible. The cumulative decay of the system ultimately leads to its collapse.

We have noted the similarities between the way that a power station 'ages' and human aging, both of which are subject to inevitable decay. But there is also a fundamental difference between them — unlike power stations and nuclear reactors, every human being forms an organic system. What distinguishes the human organism from a mechanical system is that it can activate its capacity for personal agency and — to a certain extent — take steps to cope with its own processes of decay. This ability of the human organism allows it to retard the process of decay in a way that a mechanical system cannot. This is a unique human ability, one which contemporary science has begun to uncover.

Human beings differ from all other animals in that they have the ability to combine the biological components of their make-up with the cognitive components in order to delay the decay process. While the biological–physical components are subject to the law of decay, and this process accelerates in the elderly, the components that make up a person's 'spiritual' identity can potentially grow stronger.

Our propensity to focus on the spiritual dimension of life, especially in the advanced stages, has long been recognized over time and across all cultures, but has rarely been directed towards the body and its needs.

On the contrary, spiritual traditions have demanded detachment from the physical, on the assumption that a preoccupation with the body and the bodily would undermine the focus on spiritual concerns.

However, what we are now discovering is that human beings constitute an integrated system capable of producing comprehensive developmental change by integrating their physical and non-physical dimensions and activating them in order to delay the inevitable decay that is the fate of every organism.

Aging is not a one-way process, tending only in the direction of wear and tear. Parallel to decline, we also have the potential for renewal. And the process by which this is achieved depends on us.

Such is the power of the human mind that it enables us to integrate our thoughts, our emotions and our physical and social functioning. In so doing, it can allow us not only to realize the full potential of the spiritual side of being human and to give our lives new meaning, as the psychologists have explained to us, but also to postpone the process of decay.

In contrast to mechanical systems that, despite all their complexity, are essentially 'simple systems' — systems that can be broken down into parts which can be dealt with separately — as an integrated entity the individual is a 'complex system', a system in which a synergetic relationship between its various parts and dimensions is essential to its continued operation.[6]

To put this another way: our functional age, quality of life and life expectancy are determined, to a large extent, by the synergy that exists between what I call our four personal dimensions — the cognitive, the emotional, the physical and the social. Taken together, they determine our functional age and our personal lifespan.

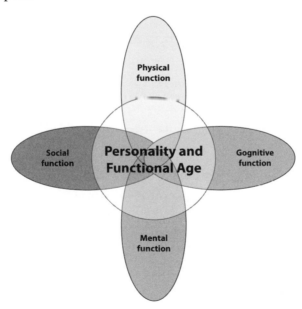

THE SYNERGETIC FACTORS DETERMING A PERSON'S FUNCTIONAL AGE

Illustration © Zvi Lanir

In the 1980s, based on his thorough documentation of patients nearing the end of their lives, family doctor and gerontologist Marian Rabinowitz put forward the then revolutionary idea that for the elderly, chronological age is not a reliable indicator of a person's health status and life expectancy. What actually determines one's state of health in old age is a combination of different 'ages' — functional age, social age, emotional age, cognitive age and biological age. For each indicator, an individual may be a different 'age'. Only when they are seen in combination does the functional age and 'personal chronology' of the individual concerned emerge.

Very few humans age uniformly across all the dimensions of their make-up; most people will be young in one component and old in others. Therefore, Rabinowitz argued, conventional definitions of 'old' and 'young' are meaningless, and he suggested abandoning the old/young dichotomy altogether.

Despite the very positive reception of Rabinowitz's book, *The Six Ages of Man and the Inner Time*,[7] by the gerontology community in Israel, his ideas were not taken up and research on this subject has progressed little beyond what Rabinowitz himself proposed.

Notwithstanding this, his ideas have substantially influenced my own research. However, while

Rabinowitz's approach was mainly therapeutic, mine is proactive and pre-emptive. My aim is to show people how they can actively manipulate their functional age and create a 'personal reserve' that will enable them to enjoy the wisdom years and postpone the infirmities of old age.

PART THREE

Enjoying the Wisdom
Years

Introduction to Part Three

The theoretical introduction to the wisdom years that I have presented in Part Two, although by no means comprehensive, is sufficient to enable us to move on to its practical implementation.

Specifically, in Part Three I focus on getting to grips with the individuation process. While both Jung and Erikson focused on the psychological aspects of this process, my contribution has been to integrate the cognitive and bio-systemic elements of the process, essential to tailoring it to the requirements of the wisdom years.

Individuation is the process which guides us in activating the three lobes of the brain discussed above in order to modify our mind maps to equip us for the wisdom years. These new maps will enable us to function as a unified system, integrating our physical, mental, emotional and social dimensions. Successfully integrating these elements will substantially influence the quality and length of our active life.

This section of the book is devoted to the implementation of the individuation process. Each of the next four chapters is dedicated to a different dimension of our human make-up, offering guidelines tailored to that particular element. However, as I have emphasized, the synergy between all four dimensions is essential to generating change. Thus, in each chapter I also discuss how the activation of a particular dimension can synergistically enhance the other three. In Chapter 16, I tackle the question of when the age of wisdom becomes 'old age'.

I end the book by reviewing my own experience of the wisdom years using the insights I have discovered through my personal journey.

Chapter 12

Mind Your Body

The individuation of our body is the natural first step in the process of personal renewal for the wisdom years. The benefits become apparent immediately, while at the same time they have the potential for long term effects on the other elements of our make-up.

The first immediate benefit is an increase in oxygen. Physical exercise is necessary for the maintenance of a healthy body. However, since exercise increases oxygen supply, it is also vital for the maintenance of a healthy brain. While the brain weighs only 2 per cent of the body, it uses up 20 per cent of the available oxygen. Most of the oxygen utilized in the brain is used for communication within the brain's internal networks, thus enabling healthy functioning of our mind maps. These processes continue to function and use oxygen even when we are at rest.

Regular physical exercise is also important for the creation and release into the brain of BDNF — brain-derived neurotrophic factor. This protein plays a major role in the health and function of neurons, in preserving the brain's elasticity and in the creation of new brain cells.[1]

Physical exercise keeps the mind alert, stimulated and challenged. This is an antidote to our natural inclination as older folk for sitting back and sinking into a lazy routine, an attitude which would in effect retire our minds.

Forming New Habits

Another major benefit is the habit-changing process which we undergo as we seek to modify our physical exercise habits. The renewal promised by the wisdom years needs a mindful change of habits. During the hectic years of maintaining a growing family and career, we may have grown used to certain habits which we no longer need. Letting go of redundant or bad habits and acquiring new ones is a difficult process, but one which is easier to begin by changing our physical routines.

When we retire, we can very easily slide into mindless, lazy habits — which require very little willpower to maintain. We may find ourselves watching TV endlessly, overeating and staying home rather than making the effort to get out and meet new people. If we continue such habits we will become bored, isolated, depressed, lonely and then simply old.

Physical exercise can be a major trigger for changing our habits, as every small step forward is visible and even measurable. The success brought by each seemingly minor achievement can inspire us to carry on.

Once our minds have experienced habit changing, our reward centres will have learned their benefits. This in turn will enhance our readiness to acknowledge and change other, less tangible habits

Experts in this field differentiate between 'regular habits' and 'key habits'.[2] This chapter focuses on physical exercise as our primary key habit, modifications to which can trigger a chain reaction of habit changes.

No one would disagree that incorporating an appropriate exercise routine into one's life has positive physical effects. However, it triggers changes in other habits, both physical and nonphysical. People who make a habit of mindfully activating their body begin to eat healthier and are motivated to stop smoking and improve their sleeping habits. They dare to try new things in life and become more resilient in times of crisis. They end up becoming more mindful, both of themselves and others.

How do we change our habits? The process starts with a cue — a trigger which automatically stimulates our mind to activate a habit. Once we receive the cue, we begin performing the activity as a given, habitual routine. We then get the reward which our brain craves.

This reward is generated by the reward centre in our brains, which creates pleasurable feelings linked to certain actions.[3] This in turn influences our routines and habits, as it strengthens certain behaviours and makes it more likely that we will repeat them. Reactivating the neurons in the brain's reward centre generates a rush of the neural agent dopamine. Dopamine makes us feel good, so we want to repeat the process.

Businesses know how to trigger the habit loop so that we get hooked on their products. McDonald's restaurants, for example, are designed and run so that a particular habit loop is implanted in our brains. All McDonald's branches are designed identically, both architecturally and internally. The employees all speak the same product 'language' and offer the same meals. Taken together, these elements form a permanent cue which triggers eating habits around food which is also specifically designed to provide immediate gratification. This enjoyment triggers our reward centres, making us want more of the product, thus completing our unconscious habit loop.

Understanding how the habit loop functions will help us acquire new habits and rid ourselves of harmful old habits.

We can start acquiring more useful habits by activating the brain's frontal lobe while at the same time contemplating the new habit we wish to embrace. Having considered this new habit, try to determine an appropriate cue.

For instance, if you want to start your day with a run, try putting your running shoes and clothing next to the bed. This is the first step, which will prompt the mind to make running a habit — even when you would rather do anything but running. To overcome this internal opposition, you must proceed to the second step, which involves performing the routine activity (in this case, getting up and running) every day, in the same sequence. The third step involves the reward, where your mind urges you to repeat the exercise. To reach this final step, you should strive to make small steps at a time, thereby achieving results that are tangible and measurable. For instance, if running is the new habit you're trying to master, measure the distance or speed covered today and compare it with yesterday's achievements. If you persevere, your mind will continue to seek the reward offered by the endorphins released during your daily run.

For most people, persistence is the biggest stumbling block when trying to master a new habit. The lack of an immediate reward is the reason why so many people who sign up for the gym drop out after only a few weeks. However, those who manage to persist through the habit threshold continue, as they look forward to the pleasure provided by the brain's reward centre during training and afterwards. My gym manager told me that he has a 180-day rule: most people who sign up don't last beyond 180 days. But those who persevere past this point will often continue their training for many years.

In time, the steps on the habit loop become interconnected: cueing, routine exercise and the reward experienced in the brain strengthen each other and function in tandem. Things get to the stage that once the cue appears, a strong craving for the reward creates an addiction.

I used this process to get myself to practise yoga every morning. In time, it became a permanent habit which I now can't imagine living without. Routine is the key. I get up every day at the same time (5.30 am, winter and summer) and perform the same routine in the same order, using the same mat, in front of the same window overlooking the park.

In the beginning, I had to concentrate on every exercise but, with time, doing them became automatic. My mind and body now perform the yoga exercises automatically, without the need for conscious thought. They've become a habit which my mind and body look forward to. I won't easily give up these magic 10 minutes of my morning workout and the pleasure they give me.

Starting with the Body

Individuation requires us to be aware of the connections between thoughts, feelings and actions. Instilling this awareness starts with mindfulness for our bodies. This is another reason I recommend beginning the process of personal renewal with individuation of the body. The hardship and effort involved in stretching the limbs and muscles offer excellent opportunities for training our awareness of what we are doing, feeling and thinking in various states of activity, as well as at rest.

When you focus and persevere at a given task, you will, in time, notice that your body has a personality of its own. It too has good days and bad days. Its behaviour and mood can change from day to day. At times, your body will inform you that you should 'let it go' or 'take it easy'. On other days it is energetic and raring to go. You must teach yourself to be sensitive to the different 'moods' of your body and love it. This will improve your attentiveness and sensitivity in other areas of your life.

If you have never engaged in any kind of regular exercise or sport, you may be wondering which to choose and how to make a start. The large variety on offer lets you choose what you can afford and what will suit you best. A combination of activities is probably a good idea. Any physical exercise is good for both mind and soul. However, some have extra benefits for the mind, such as yoga, Pilates, biking, swimming, running and walking. A combination of these modes is even more beneficial.

Be sure to include aerobic exercise in your routine, as it increases oxygen uptake as well as the heart rate, supplying the oxygen required for our body and brain. Power training is also important for the maintenance of our skeleton and muscles, but must be done in moderation. As we get older, it should be used to maintain muscle mass and prevent bone depletion rather than to develop a muscular physique.

For older people, high intensity training should last no longer than 20–45 minutes. Longer or more intensive sessions increase the risk of injury. I suggest that you choose exercise routines which utilize various muscles simultaneously, thus distributing the strain and enabling you to enjoy your body as an integrated system.

If you are interested in belonging to a gym or health club, I recommend that you join one which employs coaches who will teach you how to perform these exercises correctly. I have found that many trainers are not aware of older people's needs in this area.

It is important that you always pay attention to your body during training. I have taught myself to listen to my body, and I stop when the pleasure I normally take in physical exercise turns to pain. Using this distinction, I build up to this limit and do not go past it. It is important that part of your training be done in a group setting. For older exercisers, being part of a group is encouraging. And it has the added bonus of extending one's social circle.

Physical exercise should not be limited to the gym. Make sure that you have enough equipment at home so that you can integrate exercise breaks into your daily routine. Equipment like small weights, rubber bands, a fit ball and pressure rings are not expensive. Just make sure that you are trained to use them properly.

While physical exercise is very important, continuing to perform routine tasks at home is valuable, too. You may not have cleaned, cooked or washed dishes when younger; you may also have chosen to hire specialists for small repair tasks. I suggest that you change these habits by routinely seeking every opportunity to mindfully perform these activities. They promote fine motor coordination between your mind and your fingers, which is important for maintaining the flexibility of brain functions as we age. Giving them up may compromise the mind's alertness and flexibility.

So, when something breaks, don't rush to the expert. Use the opportunity to train your brain and to activate unfamiliar mind and body coordination skills. Trying it yourself is worthwhile even if the plumber, carpenter or bicycle repairer can do the job better and faster.

Computer games provide another opportunity for enjoying a challenge and building your achievement levels while improving fine motor hand–eye coordination. So do join in when your grandchildren want to play computer games with you, even though you know there is no chance of beating them!

If you've danced in the past, and even if you haven't, now is the time to put on your dancing shoes. Dancing improves flexibility and can prevent balance problems and falls. In addition, learning new dance moves strengthens agility through the combined activation of the three lobes of the brain. When you dance, you use your left lobe to follow the directions you're receiving from your teacher or partner; your right lobe takes charge of the emotions and imagination inherent in dancing; and you are teaching your rear lobe to perform the dance steps instinctively. Dancing offers an ideal opportunity to activate the physical, mental, emotional and social components of your make-up in an integrated manner.

Changing Nutritional Habits

Having acquired the habit of physical exercise, you will instinctively seek to improve your nutrition. People who exercise regularly are more aware of what they eat, how much they eat and how they consume their food than those who take little exercise. Nutrition, like moving our body, influences our brain. The unhealthy foods we consume and the healthy alternatives we push aside hurt our brains as well as well as our bodies.

Overeating gives us a heavy feeling, reducing our ability to act and think. While sugar gives us an energy boost, we soon feel tired again. Some foods are more important for us as we get older, as they counteract the damage done to our aging bodies and minds by free radicals (chemicals created in oxygenated cells). Free radicals cause cellular imbalance, are harmful to our DNA and trigger destructive chemical reactions. Foods rich in antioxidants like vitamins C and E, selenium and the preservative BHT can block free radical activity, or at least slow it down. Neuron regeneration is aided by the consumption of flavonoids (pigments found in blueberries and bitter chocolate, for example), Omega-3 (abundant in salmon, avocado and walnuts) and moderate drinking of red wine. On the other hand, consumption of saturated fat harms neural growth. The physical act of chewing, as opposed to consuming foods with a creamy texture, also helps to maintain brain cell health and regeneration.

While some studies have suggested a connection between nutrition and the emotions, definitive results have proved elusive. But who could argue with sentiments like: 'Eating chocolate can put you in a good mood' or 'Wine brings people closer.'

Discussing changes in eating habits raises the question of how we let go of negative habits. Adding new foods to our diet is less of a problem than freeing ourselves from reliance on unhealthy foods. We can overcome such addictions by retaining the cue and reward routine, but adding a new activity between them. This way we can turn the negative habit into a positive one.

To beat the bad habit, we must first identify the three elements of the habit loop which we want to dump. Having identified them, we can now consider how to replace old routines with new ones.

At one time, I was in the habit of taking a break after several hours of work and going down to the local coffee shop, where I would order coffee and cake. I thought that my sweet tooth was the culprit. Even though I knew that sugar was detrimental to my health, I couldn't break the sugar addiction supported by those daily morning outings for coffee and cake.

My road to freedom appeared when I began investigating the rewards I got from this habit. Having explored the issue mindfully, I concluded that it provided a break from the intensive mental work that occupied me. Walking to the coffee shop gave me this break, as well as the opportunity for short but enjoyable conversations with other customers.

This analysis led me to understand that my coffee habit resulted from the need for respite, and for human contact. I craved temporary distraction and social interaction, and both these needs were met by my regular visits to the coffee shop. Once I identified my hidden needs, I could redesign my habit. While I still visit the coffee shop every morning, I now order only sugar-free coffee and do without the cake.

My new routine didn't succeed immediately. I was sometimes tempted to order cake with my coffee. Even now, when the cake has been replaced by a delicious sandwich, I sometimes allow myself to order cake instead as a treat. However, I am no longer addicted to my morning sugar habit. I understand the cue and provide myself with a reward, even if I occasionally succumb to my original temptation.

I've gone into some detail in this discussion of ditching old habits and forming new ones, here within the context of physical exercise and nutrition. I suggest these are the first areas where we should start the process of change. The methods we have learned in these areas will prove useful when we apply the individuation process to the other dimensions of our make-up.

Chapter 13

Harnessing Our Brain Power

The human brain can activate two types of thinking — subconscious and conscious. Most of the time we are controlled by our subconscious thinking processes, and for good reason. More than 90 per cent of our reactions and behavioural habits are activated by the brain's subconscious thinking mechanism. It saves us time and brain energy.

Your subconscious thinking mode is at play when you drive. When you learned how to drive, you had to solve new and unfamiliar problems, which required conscious reflection. Now that you are an experienced driver, your driving is almost automatic, requiring very little conscious thinking. Your brain has acquired a 'driving mind map' and your responses to road conditions are controlled by your 'auto-pilot', which is chiefly operated by the rear lobe of the brain. When the 'auto-pilot' is turned on, the frontal lobes can relax, enabling them to switch readily to a meandering, subconscious mode of thinking. This in turn can lead your mind obsessively from one subject to another — and worse, from one worry to another. This type of thinking has been named 'monkey thinking' — because it is jumpy, messy and unruly.

However, if you are to successfully complete the individuation process for the wisdom period of your life, your conscious thinking mode needs to undergo comprehensive activation. Only in this way will you be able to examine and reframe the thoughts, reactions and habits you acquired during adulthood. It is your capacity for active, conscious thinking that will enable you to cope with the complex issues you will have to deal with at this stage of your life. This can be done by activating all the three lobes of the brain simultaneously, gradually creating new mind maps appropriate for the wisdom period.

This is a continuous process, not a one-time event after which you can return to 'normal' thinking. Rather, it should become your primary mode of thinking, and you should work at maintaining it.

You can create conscious thinking patterns and adopt a conscious lifestyle by becoming aware of your daily habits. Once you are aware of them, you can decide if those are habits you want to keep in your newly motivated life, where change is a constant. Furthermore, it is important to activate your conscious thinking to encompass all aspects of your life — physical, emotional and social. This will in turn enable you to pose and answer abstract and spiritual questions regarding your life's meaning and purpose.

During adulthood, most of us were faced with day-to-day pressures and worries. The need to quickly switch between tasks, or multitask, made it harder for us to focus on active, conscious thinking, which requires more time and brain energy. But now, post-retirement, we can and should allow ourselves to let go of such pressures, including the habit of responding quickly to the multiple demands on our attention. This will give us the time and mind energy we need to focus on active, conscious thinking.

As we make the effort to stay within our active, conscious thinking mode, random, wandering thoughts will distract us less and less. If we don't take the initiative here, our minds are likely to be overtaken by such thoughts — even more than before, as we now have more time to entertain such subconscious thinking. When wandering thoughts take control, they negatively affect our mind and our mood. This engenders a pessimistic outlook which lowers our self-esteem and happiness.

In 2010, *Science* magazine published an article titled 'A Wandering Mind is an Unhappy Mind' which described the results of an international study of 2250 volunteers, aged 18–88.[1] It used a cellphone application to record the participants' levels of happiness in relation to their activities and thoughts at the time they reported them. The study found that their thoughts were wandering 46.9% of the time, regardless of what they were doing. It also found a negative correlation between reported levels of happiness and wandering thoughts: the more wandering thoughts, the less contentment.

Managing our active, conscious thinking involves a cyclic, three-phase process which utilizes the three lobes of our brain. The process starts by activating the right lobe, triggering a kind of 'conversation' between the right and the left lobes and allowing our thinking to become more complex and sophisticated. Finally, we activate the rcar lobe, working in tandem with our two frontal lobes.

What follows are some practical guidelines for deliberately activating our conscious thinking mode.

The First Phase

We trigger the right lobe of our brain by activating our senses and feelings when we experience new, unfamiliar situations. What is meant by 'senses' and 'feelings' in this context? We are all very familiar with the uncontrolled emotions which flood us when we are overwhelmed by anger, fear or unexpected surges of love and sexual desire. These responses are very different from what we sense and feel when we encounter issues and situations which we do not fully understand.

'Feeling' and 'sensing' both originate in the right lobe, while 'emotion' originates in our limbic brain.[2] Emotion activates excitement, while sense and feeling activate awareness. Such awareness triggers our right lobe to choose a conscious thinking cycle.

You can teach yourself to become mindful of your ability to sense and feel. To do so, first try to become aware of the difference between what you feel when subject to a powerful emotion and what you experience when confronted by a confusing or previously unknown situation.

The distinction between feeling and sensing is negligible. I might say, 'I feel uncomfortable with my own answers'; or, 'I'm sensing that this whole subject is being ignored.' The main verb carries the same meaning in both these sentences, and either can stir our right lobe into action.

Such feelings and sensations become especially apparent when we are in a state of mindful awareness of what we are experiencing in the present moment. The benefits of mindfulness for reduction of tension, anxiety and stress are well known. However, in this context, we are wanting to explore the way it triggers and influences the right lobe of the brain.

Mindfulness can be applied to whatever we do. It enables us to be aware of what is happening to us while we are experiencing it. It also helps us note what is eluding us if our thoughts are wandering.

There is a synergetic loop between our ability to maintain a mindful presence and our ability to sense and feel. The more fully we are present in the 'here and now', the more we become aware of sensing and feeling what we didn't before.

Personally, I have gained numerous insights while maintaining a mindful awareness of this kind, a state which has enabled me to become aware of the sensations and feelings which the insights triggered within me. In fact, this book is largely based on insights I gained about my own feelings and emotions in this way. It includes numerous examples illustrating the effects that this process and the insights that accompanied it had on me.

You can train yourself to be mindful of your sensations and feelings, as with any other aspect of who you are. At first, you will succeed only intermittently. However, if you persevere, you will gradually improve this skill. As your ability improves, you will be able to appreciate and differentiate the various nuances and levels of your awareness.

In addition to these personal benefits, I have found that these skills have improved my ability to notice when others are at the mercy of wandering thoughts. I have also learned to ask relevant questions which can steer them towards active thinking, helping them overcome their lack of patience and set ways of thinking. If you can gain these skills, you may find that you are more interesting to others as well to yourself, becoming a self-enriching person.

These benefits carry their own intrinsic value. But beyond this, they also enable the activation of the second phase of the 'active thinking' cycle.

The Second Phase

Thinking about the meaning of what one has sensed and felt triggers a 'conversation' between the right and left lobes of the frontal brain. The right lobe 'queries' the left lobe about the meaning of what you have experienced but don't yet understand. This conversation between the two frontal lobes will provide new levels of understanding about the initial insight.

When you have a new insight, it is important to name it as a concept. Conceptualization serves three complementary purposes. First, naming the concept, in itself, is a learning process which enriches us with new understanding of its meaning. Second, naming the concept ensures that our brain will not forget it. And third, once we have consciously named the concept in question, the insights and knowledge we have acquired in a specific context are translated to a higher level of abstraction. The abstraction of the concept enables us to use it to interpret similar situations and contexts.[3]

For example, I devised the concept of 'the age of wisdom' as the result of a multi-step process. First, I allowed myself to become aware of ('sense and feel') my reactions after being told that I was officially old. Once I conceptualized what I sensed and felt, the various meanings of this new stage of my life became apparent. After giving a name to the concept, I began to see that it had implications and significance far beyond myself.

The process of teasing out the various meanings of 'the age of wisdom' enabled me to develop other, related concepts. Together, they created a rich new perceptual space — a vital antithesis to conventional concepts of aging which present later life as an ongoing, inevitable decline.

This new set of concepts will serve you well on your own journey to discover the wisdom years. They will guide you through your personal individuation process, but only after you have infused them with content and meaning relevant to your own life.

Patience and perseverance are needed for acquiring the skill of developing new insights and concepts. Having achieved this, your wandering thoughts will no longer rule your mind. On the contrary, they will trigger significant new associations, not trivial ones. This will enable you to create new connections between a variety of concepts, thus enriching your insights.

Each of us can develop ways of harnessing our free-ranging thoughts for good. I prefer to allow my brain to wander and reflect while I am walking in the park or on the beach, playing with my grandchildren, taking a hot shower or settling down for a good night's sleep. Our minds know how to utilize relaxed settings such as these to mull over new ways of dealing with unsolved problems.

The Third Phase

The wisdom years require that we change not only our thinking, but also our behaviour and habits. We need to create new habits which fit our new circumstances. At the same time, we need to rid ourselves of old habits which no longer serve us and may be harming us.

As we have seen in Chapter 10, the rear lobe plays a major role in creating these changes in habits. We need to mindfully integrate the activation of the frontal lobes with the rear lobe, the part of the brain responsible for our automatic functions and routine behaviour.

To succeed in the individuation process, it is essential that we teach ourselves how to activate the integration of the three lobes of our brains, consciously and mindfully, and make this process a habit. During our earlier life stages, we thought, felt and acted without reflecting on the brain mechanisms which enable these functions. Now we must become familiar with the processes our brains undergo. Only in this way can we steer and channel them purposefully in everything we choose to do — or refrain from doing.

The habit of mindful activation of our brain needs constant practice so that it becomes an intrinsic part of who we are. We must repeat it again and again, in different situations and with the appropriate adjustments. Gradually, the synaptic connections between the lobes will create a new 'habit mind map'.

Once this way of thinking and acting becomes a habit, it will no longer require so much 'brain power'. Then we will be able to free up our minds to cope with other fundamental changes we want to create in our lives.

Chapter 14

Finding Happiness and Tackling Depression

So far, we have examined our feelings and sensations and how they can prompt active thinking. It is also important to consider emotions like happiness, sadness, fear and depression, their effects on us in later life and how we can best understand and cope with them.

Happiness in the wisdom years can be characterized as a feeling of well-being — a conscious state of living in peace with ourselves and our personal circumstances. It is an awareness that life is good despite the presence of hardship, poverty, illness and suffering. Happiness in the wisdom years means knowing how to accept the imperfect and find perfection within it. It requires an acceptance of the changes that affect us as we age, of the often distressing physical symptoms of old age and, finally, of the inevitability of death.

There is a profound connection between the ability to feel this kind of happiness and our ability to be mindfully present in the here and now in a way that embraces all four dimensions of our make-up.

I've shown how mindful presence can be the catalyst for active thinking. It can also be the trigger for happiness during the wisdom age of our lives.

A New Kind of Happiness

Actively seeking ways to integrate the physical, emotional, cognitive and social elements of our make-up enables us to achieve a type of happiness which was almost unknown to us when we were younger.

As we become aware of the limited time we have left, our ability to feel happy is paradoxically enhanced rather than curtailed. At first, the ever-present knowledge of the end of our lives seems like bad news. Gradually, however, we can discover its positive implications by gaining a clearer understanding of what is truly important for us in life. As Samuel Johnson put it: 'When a man knows he is to be hanged in a fortnight, it concentrates his mind wonderfully.' When people realize that their time is limited, they are in a good position to gain a clearer understanding of what is important to them and take steps to turn their desires into reality.

The major life events which made us happy when we were younger are not hard to remember: graduating, getting married, the birth of our children, gaining a sought-after job, or having a holiday in a magical location.

However, during the wisdom years, it isn't the big things which necessarily make us happy. Happiness can be found in the everyday: the first sip of morning coffee, a conversation with our spouse, having friends for dinner or playing with the grandchildren. You may already have enjoyed such simple pleasures as these in earlier times. However, now they provide a new dimension of enjoyment and meaning which you might easily have missed out on during your overburdened adult years. The mindful presence which comes your way during this final individuation process will make you more attentive to the events and moments of everyday life which bring a quiet contentment.

Anyone who has experienced this kind of happiness will find it both satisfying and rewarding. We should not be slow to express our gratitude for this new gift, both to ourselves and to others around us.

The happiness that marks the wisdom years is not necessarily without times of sadness. Happiness and sadness are not exclusive opposites, but can co-exist within us. A violin player can feel uplifted while playing a very sad melody. Happiness during the wisdom years is dependent on our ability to accept the complementary contrasts inherent in the human condition.

Coping with Mood Swings and Depression

During the first few months after retirement, one faces a considerable risk of depression or just an attack of 'the blues'. Human beings need to feel significant in some way and have tangible goals to maintain a sense of self-worth. Without such aspirations, we question the meaning and purpose of our lives.

Overcoming this potential crisis is a substantial issue within the individuation process. Successfully coping with it, both intellectually and emotionally, heralds the growth of a new, integrated personality.

Those who fail to cope may find themselves subject to ongoing episodes of depression. This can cause sufferers to exaggerate minor failures and unpleasant events, and to minimize their own successes and strong points. Positive events are dwarfed by negative ones, good memories become blurred and bad ones are repeated over and over.

I've met people whose lives took a downhill slide when they retired. They began to burrow into the hurts and failures they had suffered in the past. Their life stories became narratives of misery and they were full of guilt, directed both at themselves and others. Such folk complain so loudly that their grievances seem to have taken over their lives. Instead of being grateful for what they *do* have — which could enrich their lives and provide them with new meaning — they constantly focus on what they *don't* have.

Fortunately, however, studies of happiness in later life show that such people are in the minority. In one study, Laura Carstensen of Stanford University asked volunteers aged 18 to 90+ to keep diaries detailing their feelings and emotional states in various situations. She found that older people expressed fewer negative emotions, dealt better with personal criticism and achieved a healthier balance between happiness and sadness.[1] The study showed that while for younger people five positive scores were needed to outweigh a single negative score, older participants needed only two positives for every negative, as they were more able to focus on the positive aspects.

However, such findings do not mean that older people live in a feel-good haze of passive thinking. On the contrary, fMRI scans of their brains showed that older people who interpret life in positive terms use their front brains more actively.[2] Active thinking enables them to cope better with negative emotions, to accept distressing things as they happen, to relate to injustice with compassion rather than despair, and to cope better with emotionally loaded arguments. To these findings I would add that active thinking protects their minds from being taken over by anxious, wandering thoughts — ruminations which originate in the rear lobe of the brain and are one of the major causes of low mood and depression.

If we are to believe the medical and geriatric establishment, antidepressants and psychogeriatric drugs are the main channels for treating depression in older people. I am not opposed to using medication for difficult cases. At the same time, I want to stress that we can — and need — to identify the problems involved ourselves and deal with them on our own. We can treat ourselves cognitively and mentally when we recognize the initial stages of depressive states. Early diagnosis and action can prevent the deterioration which will eventually cause dependence on medication and psychogeriatric treatment regimes.

Depression has its own stages of development. The first stage is characterized by low mood and anxieties which flood the mind. If we don't confront these feelings at this stage, they are likely to grow stronger and trigger further negative thoughts: 'I can no longer do what I used to do in the past; it's getting worse and worse'; 'Enough, it's too late'; 'There's no point to trying again'; 'There's nothing to live for any more.' If we continue in this vein, our mind develops a depressive mind map, which produces increasingly negative thoughts. Depression becomes a habit which overwhelms our mind and is hard to rid ourselves of.

To prevent this outcome, we must take active measures to cope with low moods when they first occur. Such moods can appear when something irritates us, when we find ourselves alone during the holidays, when we become sick, or when we experience sad feelings for no apparent reason. We can also experience chronic sleeplessness and nightmares which cause us to relive painful memories by replaying wounding failures from the past. We need to learn when and why these 'low periods' attack us and rehearse ways of escaping or avoiding them.

To differentiate between the various types of depressive episode, and cope with them, we should be employing the mindfulness lessons we have already learned. At first, it will be hard to differentiate between the different forms of depression. However, if you continue to be attentive, you will learn to recognize and analyze them, to find the specific reason for each episode and deal with it accordingly.

Mindful Breathing

The right way of breathing is vital in such situations. I have already discussed the importance of breathing for oxygen transfer to our brain and to enhance our capacity for active thinking. Breathing is likewise essential for coping with recurring low moods and depression.

The effect of our breathing is bi-directional, since any mental state influences our breathing. When we are relaxed, our breathing will naturally be deep and slow, and will flow effortlessly. When we are fearful or anxious, our breath becomes choppy, shallow and rapid. During our adult life, we were faced with many situations which were tense, anxious, stressful or fearful. These affected our breathing, which became tense in response — typically rapid, shallow and fragmented.

Our lungs can transport up to 4 litres (1 gallon) of air during the breathing cycle (inhaling and exhaling).

However, an average person breathing normally will utilize only half a litre (0.13 gallons) of air per breath. We are bound to have acquired some bad breathing habits by the time we reach the wisdom years.

Shallow breathing, which fails to supply us with enough oxygen, causes tiredness, lowered energy and even bad moods. On the other hand, when we breathe deeply and slowly we inhale more oxygen, potentially enhancing our physical health and mental abilities. Breathing deeply and mindfully can also stave off depression and make us happier and more vibrant individuals.

It is also important to slow our breathing. The process of absorbing oxygen and releasing CO_2 takes time. When we breathe quickly, we are not giving our lungs and bodies the time necessary for optimal absorption of oxygen and evacuation of CO_2 and other toxins.

Speaking personally, once I acquired the habit of breathing slowly and deeply my breathing habits were improved by regular yoga sessions. It is not difficult to make slow breathing a habit, even without a discipline like yoga. If you persevere, the volume of air entering and leaving your lungs can reach the desired 4 litres, multiplying the circulation of oxygen in your lungs by a factor of eight.

Our way of breathing and our levels of awareness and feeling are interconnected. When we take full, slow breaths we subdue the angry, pressured, anxious thinking patterns established during our earlier lives. Then we can turn our relaxed attention inwards, focusing on ourselves. If you can train yourself to breathe deeply and relax your body, even in tense and stressful situations, you will find that it will help you let go of negative emotions.

Take advantage of any opportunity you have to breathe mindfully. This will remind you that your happiness is in your own hands and can accompany you anywhere, whatever the circumstances. At night, when you find yourself reliving painful memories and worries flood in, turn your attention to your breathing. Take deep, long and slow breaths. By concentrating on them, you will push away the negative thoughts and enjoy a peaceful sleep.

As we age, personal losses and major life crises can be 'legitimate' causes for depression: the death of a spouse or close friend, loneliness, a serious medical problem — especially one that makes us dependent on others. These things can overshadow the positive aspects of our lives and make us feel hopeless. We have all encountered people who don't know how to handle these crises and describe their lives as meaningless.

In such situations, the coping methods outlined here may be insufficient to restore our inner balance. To deal with them, we need to conscript the physical, intellectual, mental and social dimensions of our make-up and integrate them into a new, robust whole. This will give us the multi-dimensional perspective we need to escape a potentially destructive situation. This new perspective can help us devise new ways to recover our equilibrium and will to live, despite the difficult situations in which we will inevitably find ourselves in our later years.

Chapter 15

Resetting Relationships

The personal transformation that proceeds admission to the wisdom years leads us to rediscover our inner self and to redefine our needs. These changes affect our expectations of the people around us — spouses, families, friends and community.

During the individuation process, we are in a permanent dialogue with ourselves. However, to maintain this inner dialogue, we must also begin a new dialogue with our 'significant others'. Both dialogues complement and enhance each other.

Intimate Relationships

Retirement poses new questions for the relationship between spouses and partners.

We need to take a fresh look at each other's new needs and expectations, over a wide spectrum of issues. These include exploring new expressions of partnership and intimacy, new ways to fill our time, and even deciding how to share our domestic space and household chores.

Aging brings a qualitative change in the way we express our love. When we were young, the peak of intimacy was embodied in sex. Now we can express it in many other ways — through friendship, tenderness, affection and the mature wisdom we discover within ourselves. These all influence the kind of intimacy we will be able to maintain in later life.

When we were young and in love (in the conventional sense), we tended to see our beloved as a reflection of ourselves. We ignored the elements of their personality which did not fit the image we had of ourselves, exemplifying the old saying that 'love is blind.'

The individuation process enables us to open our eyes and see our life partner in a new way. As we change by recognizing that our respective needs are not in fact identical, we enrich our love and our life together. We come to see it as a love between two separate, unique souls who complement each other.

Retirement changes the position of both men and women within a relationship. Men's status has been largely defined by their position in the workplace, while women's status and self-esteem has been tied to their activities in the home and relationships within the family. Hence retirement is generally a more daunting prospect for men. In any case, retirement often upsets the equilibrium that had been maintained in a couple's earlier years.

For example, one of my friends confided to me, albeit with some exaggeration, how she feels in this new situation. She observed that since his retirement, her husband doesn't know what to do with himself. She added that he's 'bothering' her all the time, making her feel that he's 'driving her crazy'.[1]

As the old equilibrium has been upset, your spouse may unconsciously attempt to retrieve it by steering you back into your old role. Part of the individuation process for this stage of life involves consciously facing up to this issue. You will learn how to gradually rebalance the relationship by finding new roles for both partners. These roles should be based on an acceptance of the need to create expectations of each other that are grounded in reality. When we were young and in love, we did not doubt that our spouse would fulfil all our emotional needs. We then felt disappointed and hurt when this didn't happen. Now we need to realize that such expectations are not realistic, and indeed never were. We must create a new equilibrium that takes account of our new roles and the changed sources of our self-esteem.

Hopefully, an open and frank discussion of these changes and their implications will result in a new kind of intimacy and a new 'marriage contract' which will take account of each other's newly discovered needs.

Family Relationships

Having faced up to the issues with our partner, we need to consider how our new situation will affect our wider family.

It is important to make our extended family members aware of how we want to live in this new period of our lives. We should also make it clear that we expect them to respect our wishes.

Don't repress the legitimate expectations you have of your adult children. I frequently hear people saying resentfully: 'If I don't expect anything of my children, I won't be disappointed.' In fact, repressed expectations can readily turn into feelings of frustration, cause passive–aggressive behaviour and provoke angry responses from both sides.

In earlier generations, the 'contract' implicitly agreed between parents and children contained a number of assumptions. While the adults were raising the children, the children were dependent on them and were expected to obey the rules they set down. Once the parents retired, these roles were reversed. But now, retirement no longer implies that the older generation will be infirm and dependent. Since dependency is no longer the basis of the relationship, a new foundation is required.

While most of us don't want to cut our ties with family, we need to clearly establish new boundaries that will enable our personal development. Following conventional expectations, your family may now view you at least in part as a 'babysitter', while you are building a different identity for yourself. The individuation process will bring you back to your family with a different mindset, one which will help you manage newly emerging issues.

You will need to learn to steer clear of the tensions inherent in every extended family. For example, you will need to learn how to deal with your children's not infrequent requests for money — while at the same time they insist that you not meddle in their financial decisions.

These kinds of issues can easily undermine family relationships. However, the wisdom which you are in the process of acquiring will help you devise new coping methods, which in turn will enable you to redefine your relationships on a new basis.

Separation without detachment and involvement without meddling are the keys to redefining these relationships. Separation represents the space and freedom you need for your personal evolution. It should be clear to you and the rest of the family that you don't need anyone to tell you whether what you do is 'appropriate'. However, you should use your newfound wisdom in applying separation without emotional detachment. Such an approach will bring new life to your extended family relationships, rather than undermining them.

One of the benefits of individuation is acquiring a deep knowledge of one's inner self. Having set out on this path, you will be well placed to strike a productive balance between your own sense of self and your interaction with family members.

The responsibility of finding these new pathways is yours. Don't expect your family members to take the initiative. How you act when faced with challenging situations is how you will pave the way ahead. Along the route, you may find yourself becoming the one who handles conflict and solves problems.

The second principle, involvement without meddling, is just as important for redefining your relationships. Involvement is an expression of interest, care and consideration about what is happening in the lives of others. It lets your significant others know just how much they mean to you, that they are not alone in facing the issues life throws up, and that you care.

Meddling on the other hand is perhaps best defined as interfering with other people's business. If nothing else, your awareness of your changed position within the family circle should dissuade you from intruding in your children's lives. Letting go will enable you to deal with family tensions and disputes in a non-judgmental manner, while still being fully involved in family affairs.

Disputes and disagreements are commonplace in extended families, each side convinced that their solution is the correct one. Once you've let go of meddling, you are well placed to become an arbiter who comes up with a creative, third solution that no one had considered. With your life experience and accumulated wisdom, you are in a good position to maintain empathy for all family members equally, always with their best interests at heart.

Interacting with your grandchildren has many benefits. The most obvious one is your contribution of time: you free up their parents' time, and the grandkids enjoy the release of being (temporarily) free of parental discipline. Another obvious benefit is the mutual enjoyment experienced by grandparents and grandchildren who get to spend time with each other.

However, interaction with grandchildren has a further benefit for people undergoing the individuation process of the wisdom years. Engaging with your grandchildren through playing and talking will reveal new ways of enriching the process which you are undergoing. As you observe closely how they think, play and do things, you will learn from the evidence of their thought processes — their natural use of emotional, preformal thinking to grasp the essence of anything new they encounter, as well as the way they project non-trivial associations to build and enrich their internal world.[2]

Do it soon, before they grow up! School undermines their innocent preformal thinking and imaginative engagement with things, seeking to replace it with formal thinking.

Friends and Friendships

Doctors and psychologists stress the benefits of maintaining friendships and relationships as we age. These enhance our well-being and longevity, while preventing loneliness. The individuation process enables you to be more selective in this area. You can let go of superficial friendships while investing only in those which are important to you.

It is often said that older people are less capable of maintaining friendships than the young, and even less adept at initiating new relationships. However, research shows that this belief is ill-founded. Apparently, our emotional–social intelligence (ESI) improves as we age.[3] Emotional competency tends to decrease between young adulthood and middle adulthood, but increases again in later life.[4]

ESI is a holistic combination of wisdom, emotion and social skills. When we go through the individuation process, we become more aware of what we are looking for in friendships. In addition, we become more sensitive to the feelings and needs of our friends. The new cognitive competence we gain as we age increases our social skills. We become more generous, considerate and forgiving, and more able to let go of anger.

These skills can help us renew friendships which had been cut short because of past hurts. Our new sensitivity to social situations enables us to reconsider the personal significance of these friendships, allowing us to realize that we truly miss our former friends.

We also gain the ability to assess whether a new acquaintance can become a friend, and then initiate such friendships. We now possess the social tools to befriend people across different age brackets. Such friendships will enrich us as we come to share part of their world, widening the scope of our interests, horizons and involvement in society.

Considering all these potential benefits, I was not surprised by the results of a series of studies on 'social expertise' conducted by the psychologist Thomas Hess. Hess found that social expertise reaches a peak in later life.[5]

Sadly, it seems that few older people make use of these abilities. Many tend to shut themselves indoors. They avoid getting out in the evenings, claiming tiredness as an excuse. Avoidance gradually becomes a habit. Many elderly folk simply sink into their armchairs, giving up anything which requires moving out of their comfort zone.

The individuation process can help us to break the habit of social avoidance — just as we can break the habit of avoiding physical exercise. Breaking out of our physical activity and social comfort zones will do much to improve our physical and social health. As we saw in Chapter 12, it is important to start with physical activity. It will help you cope better with the tiredness and lack of motivation which cause you to fall asleep in front of the TV at 8 pm.

Another common reason for leaving our new social abilities on the shelf is the belief that older bodies are ugly, and that now we are retired we've ceased to be attractive. The media disseminates the insidious stereotype that beauty and attractiveness belong only to youth. The anti-aging industries work very hard to convince us that we must follow their prescriptions In order to maintain our 'youth'.

One of the benefits of the individuation process is that it enables us to refute these stereotypes and let them go. If we allow our personalities to shine by being interesting, surprising, and even cool and naughty, we turn out to be much more fun to be with than when we were young.

Attractiveness during the wisdom years is a different quality than that encountered in adulthood. It doesn't matter how many wrinkles we have, whether we have fatter arms as women or skinnier arms as men, and whether our hair has turned grey — or white.

Our calling card to the outer world should now be featuring our inner vitality and wisdom in large font. Our personality now becomes our greatest asset. It makes us genuinely attractive, despite the seeming 'failure of the body'.

Introducing ourselves to strangers can be an embarrassing exercise at any age. Many of us are too shy to take the first step. However, if you can overcome your diffidence, you'll be surprised at the positive response you will get. Other people your age are looking to cement new contacts just as much as you are, and younger people will also be intrigued when you approach them.

Another kind of beneficial friendship is found in books and reading, even though the relationship is distinctly one-sided. The saying 'a good book is your best friend' is only a small exaggeration. A good book can inspire your thoughts and activate your emotions even more than a human friend. In many cases, reading is an opportunity for an intimate virtual meeting with the author, who then becomes a significant other for you.

The wisdom period offers the opportunity to return to reading in the way you did as a child. Then, you were able to form intimate friendships with a book's heroes, as well as with the author, and talk to them in your wandering thoughts and dreams. This ability may have been put aside as you grew into an adult, due to overwhelming demands on your time and attention. Now you should try to recapture the experiences you enjoyed in your childhood reading. Imagine that the book was written just for you, and that the author is talking to you personally.

When I find a book which resonates with me, I often find myself noting down my comments, feelings and thoughts in the margins. As I continue reading, I sometimes get the feeling that what follows is the author's 'response' to my own reactions to earlier parts of the book. I often return to the paragraphs which I marked. I try to remember what they had meant to me when I first read them, and how my thinking has evolved since.

As the author of the book you are now reading, I hope my writing is 'talking' to you. If you are treating the book as a personal conversation with me, my efforts have been justified. I would like to think that it resonates with you, triggering thoughts and ideas and perhaps written comments of your own.

Community Relationships

Entering the wisdom years transforms the meanings of our relationships with our spouses, family, friends — and books. The process also leads us to re-evaluate the importance of community to our personal development and well-being.

Michel Follen, a Belgian demographer, has mapped the places in the world where people live substantially longer than elsewhere, marking these places in blue. Dan Buettner, journalist, researcher and author, has taken Follen's findings one step further. In 2004, he headed a National Geographic expedition tasked with investigating some of these 'blue' areas more closely, visiting Okinawa in southern Japan, the Nicoya peninsula in Costa Rica and a Seventh Day Adventist community in the suburb of Loma Linda in Los Angeles. Buettner published his findings in his book *The Blue Zones: Lessons for Living Longer from the People who've Lived the Longest.*[6]

Buettner corroborated the well-attested evidence that work, physical activity, sound nutrition, belief, optimism and a sense of meaning, as well as family and friends, all contribute to longevity. However, he also found that beyond these factors, community has a major impact on longevity. His studies showed that people who enjoy a long life are highly involved in in their communities. Human beings have an inherent need to be part of a community, which if realized contributes to their well-being.

However, communities like those described in Buettner's book are very rare. Most of us do not live in 'blue zones'. Nevertheless — and, indeed, because of this — we need to give some thought to the relationships we have with the various communities we are involved in, and to their importance for our well-being.

Among other things, the individuation process encourages us to move beyond our individual resources and look for purpose and meaning in the wider society.

During the twentieth century, many of us turned our backs on traditional communities as places to live. We sought partial substitutes in communities based around professional and hobby interests and the internet. It seems that this trend is now slowly receding. A sea change is apparent in the suburbs, rural areas and big-city neighbourhoods alike. People are trying to recapture a sense of community by frequenting local coffee shops and bars and by doing more of their shopping in neighbourhood stores. They want to meet familiar faces, not anonymous figures in crowded malls. They take a genuine interest in what is happening locally and seek ways to foster their community's identity and pride in itself.

This doesn't mean that people want to return to the all-encompassing, suffocating communities of the past. Rather, they are looking for a new kind of community — places which enable interpersonal relationships without the need to give up individual space and expression. Such communities are well suited to the needs of people on the threshold of the wisdom years. Ideally, they allow residents to fulfil a need for community activism without compromising their need to express their individuality. Individuality and social activism are complementary rather than contradictory.

Now that you've retired, you can get more involved in your local community. The skills you've acquired during the individuation process have prepared you well for this role. Being a social activist within your community will enrich you as well as your community.

There are many ways to become involved. You can initiate a volunteer project or cultural group, join one of the many not-for-profit organizations seeking to combat poverty, disability or discrimination, or become an advocate for social change.

Recent studies of post-retirement volunteers found distinct differences between the factors motivating the current generation of retired volunteers and their predecessors' motives. In previous generations, people were willing to take on whatever tasks were handed to them. They were mainly concerned to avoid loneliness and boredom, while at the same time seeking to do something positive during retirement. The current generation of volunteers are more aware of their own personal needs. They are proactive and opinionated. Before taking on a new task, they want to be convinced that their efforts will make a meaningful difference, and that they will be utilizing their personal skills and motivations. Many choose to stay away from large organizations, preferring small groups where they can be satisfied that their contribution will make a tangible difference.

The sense of community is enhanced wherever retirees return for another round of active involvement. The same is true when they initiate new businesses, or even when they return to their former workplaces.[7]

The question whether online communities are beneficial to older people is open to debate. Some commentators maintain that being part of an online community can alleviate isolation and loneliness. They argue that even superficial human contact is important in old age — 'the more the merrier'. Others argue that multiple online contacts fail to offer meaningful relationships, and that in older age quality is far more important than quantity. This has been my own experience.

Even though I have multiple online 'friends', in general I find this kind of 'friendship' disappointing. These contacts do not, for the most part, provide the meaning and satisfaction provided by a tangible face-to-face community. A live contact, without electronic mediation, allows you to be human — to look people in the eye, to pat their shoulder or give them a hug. On the other hand, some relationships which begin online can later become personal, launching meaningful new friendships.

Social and Moral Attitudes

The individuation process of the wisdom years influences our broader social and moral attitudes as well.

The American psychologist, Lawrence Kohlberg, devoted his academic career to researching moral development in humans.[8] He identified three major levels of moral development across a person's lifetime. He characterized childhood as the 'pre-conventional' level, where moral boundaries are determined by an external authority. Behaviours are considered good or bad according to whether they lead to reward or punishment. The child's actions are motivated by the need to follow instructions because of their fear of authority figures.

Adulthood is characterized by Kohlberg's second level of moral development. In adulthood, we willingly obey social norms and laws. We feel the need to behave according to these rules, not just because we are afraid of punishment, but because we recognize that their maintenance is important for promoting healthy interpersonal relationships and for the existence of a well-ordered society.

The third level of moral development — the 'post-conventional level' — develops in later life. As we age, we no longer take accepted rules for granted. Rather, we judge their validity according to our personal evaluation of each situation as we encounter it. Our newly gained maturity prompts us to re-examine the dogmas which we believed in the past according to the dictates of our conscience and our perception of fairness.

In his studies, Kohlberg found that only a minority of people attain the post-conventional stage of moral perception, even in their advanced years.

You've probably noticed the correlation between these three stages in the formation of moral attitudes and the three stages in the development of human thought (see Chapter 5): the parallel between the 'pre-conventional moral level' and the preformal thinking of childhood; between the 'conventional morality' of respect for social norms and the formal thinking of adulthood; and between the 'post-conventional moral level' and the move towards postformal thinking in later life.

Postformal thinking enables us to understand that real-life situations are complex and often contain internal contradictions. However, these contradictions frequently complement each other and need to be adroitly bridged while taking account of their underlying complexity.

The individuation journey that marks the wisdom years begins by focusing inwards. This interior focus allows us to grasp the complementary relationship between our inner and outer worlds. It provides us with a new social and moral sensitivity, which can in turn trigger a new motivation to become social activists.

At the moment, the proportion of retirees involved in social activism is very small. However, as life expectancy continues to grow, more and more people will experience the wisdom years and the awareness they bring. There is a good chance that this group will become a force which will reshape society, making it more tolerant, moderate and open to pluralism.

The 'aging' of society, now still widely considered a social and economic burden, may yet show itself to be a social and economic asset, making our communities healthier places in which to live.

Chapter 16

Delaying Old Age

Aging and old age are not the same thing. Aging is a biological phenomenon, while old age is the name given to the final period of life. A person can age without becoming 'old'.

Defining oneself as old is a state of mind which implies giving up on life. As long as we are immersed in the wisdom years, we are faced with a procession of losses — of health, spouses, friends, finances and social status. The effort involved in dealing with these crises makes it increasingly difficult to maintain the integration of the four dimensions of our make-up and our functional age. As the years pass, it becomes harder to continue the task of integration, and easier to just give up. But as long as we can successfully manage the tension between aging and 'growing old', our personal age of wisdom will endure.

Our ability to maintain this tension depends on a complex array of life issues. The first and most critical is the need to find and sustain meaning in our lives.

This question scarcely bothered us during adulthood. The meaning of life was self-evident. Finding a life partner, building and supporting a family, raising our children, finding a career and climbing up the professional ladder, gaining financial independence and securing savings, and ensuring our health and happiness — these were universally accepted as the appropriate goals for adulthood. Now most of these ambitions lie behind us. We need to redefine the meaning of our lives and set new goals. If we fail to do this, we may inadvertently turn back the clock on the wisdom years, lapsing into premature old age.

During the wisdom years, seeking the meaning of life is an ongoing endeavour. We must always be looking to set goals and fill our lives with meaning, despite the inevitable losses and decline associated with aging.

As we move further on our personal individuation journey, we become empowered to find these things within our inner selves.

Once we reach deeper into our inner selves, we realize that 'finding ourselves' requires a shift of focus. We need to shift our focus outwards, onto our significant others, family, friends and community. The dual movements resulting from this bi-directional focus, inward and outward, are complementary.

Psychiatrist and Holocaust survivor Viktor Frankl wrote about the importance of looking beyond the self: 'Being human is being always directed, and pointing, to something or someone other than oneself: to a meaning to fulfil or another human being to encounter, a cause to serve or a person to love. Only to the extent that someone is living out this self-transcendence of human existence is he truly human or does he become his true self.'[1]

During the wisdom years, we are constantly striving to become the kind of independent person that Frankl describes.

We have another important lesson to learn: how to cope with the tension between this constant focus on meaning and the need to be mindfully present in the 'here and now'.

To enjoy our wisdom years, we should strive to fully experience each moment of life, without letting our thoughts wander either back to the past or forward to the future. However, in our search for meaning and purpose, our thoughts will inevitably be directed towards the future.

This seems like a contradiction, but it really describes a spiral path. During the process of individuation, we are constantly examining and clarifying our meaning and purpose in life. To do this effectively, we need to experience them in the 'here and now'.

Abstract concepts become tangible when viewed within the context of the mindful experiences of our everyday lives. These provide us with opportunities to consider their relevance and define them more explicitly.

Our words and wishes are not enough in themselves, so we need to test them through real events. The gap between what we seek and what actually happens to us can never fully be closed. While we will face plenty of ups and downs, we should not give up living in and through the contradictions they present.

During the wisdom years, we must also learn to live with the fruitful opposition between aloneness and togetherness, or solitude and community.

While it is important to spend time with our significant others, since they share our feelings, thoughts and actions, at the same time we also need to mark out space for ourselves.

Many people confuse aloneness with loneliness. They assume that being alone makes us lonely. We can feel loneliness in the company of other people, or even within a marriage. On the other hand, we can be alone but not feel lonely. Being alone is an objective fact, while being lonely is a subjective feeling. Loneliness is sad, but if you learn how to enjoy your own company and get the most out of it, being alone will not make you feel lonely. On the contrary — if you have a variety of activities which keep you busy when you are on your own, you can experience real satisfaction and joy.

There is a positive connection between the psychological situation of being alone and the human mind's ability to be creative. We need significant others to think with, but we are more able to reach creative insights when we are alone. Also, people can develop positive feelings towards others when they are alone.

Making quality time for ourselves enables us to recharge our batteries, taking new thoughts and feelings on board before meeting again with friends and family.

We can expect that we will find ourselves alone as we get older, either as a result of the death of our spouse and close friends or because we have chosen to go our separate ways. When this happens, knowing how to deal with solitude becomes extremely important, as it helps us avoid falling into depression and despair.

In the workshops I run, I've found that many people don't know how to do this. They are afraid of being alone and facing themselves. They have a constant need to be with someone else, as being alone depresses them. To avoid this situation, they search for online 'friends', hang out in crowded malls or even try obsessively to find a new spouse.

The enjoyment of one's own company is a skill that needs to be learned. My own experience has taught me that — paradoxically — knowing how to be alone is closely related to enjoying being with others. Knowing how to be alone and be enriched by the experience can improve your ability to enjoy the company of others and the gifts that flow from such interactions. Conversely, learning to be comfortable with others improves your ability to enjoy time alone.

When you find yourself happy to spend time with others, both emotionally and mentally, you will eventually feel the need to spend time with yourself so that you can internalize what you felt when you were with them. Having reflected on these thoughts and feelings, you will want to share them. Sharing the joy these impressions brought you will enrich you, and in turn enable you to enrich your significant others. The movement between solitude and companionship can be seen as a second spiral process, one which will make your life more meaningful.

On a personal level, I can honestly say that although I live alone, I don't feel lonely. I have deeper and richer connections now with family members and friends than I used to have. I feel that our mutual relationships are closer, with more love and affection flowing in both directions.

Living alone is a personal choice — it might be right for me, but not necessarily for you. Even if you live with a spouse, it is important to make time and space for yourself within the relationship. The multi-layered potential of the relationship will only be achieved when both spouses can hold their respective needs for companionship and solitude in a fruitful equilibrium.

Many people choose to move into rest homes after they retire, even though they are capable of independent living. They mistakenly identify being alone with being lonely and can't cope with the prospect of isolation. This is true both for singles and for couples who feel that they can no longer cope with their own company.

Work and Leisure

Entering the wisdom years also enables us to recalibrate the balance between work and leisure.

In his research on attitudes to work and leisure, psychologist Mihaly Csikszentmihalyi described the following paradox: when people have spent a great deal of time working, they want to escape into leisure.[2] But when we have too much leisure time on our hands, we miss our work. A healthy person needs to maintain a balance between work and leisure while extracting the maximum benefit from both. Such a balance will make our work more productive while enriching our inner lives.

Most of us will acknowledge that it was hard to maintain this balance during our adulthood. Work was usually very demanding and pressured. Our leisure time was all too short, with increasing intrusions from work.

For many of us, the lack of balance between work and leisure during our adult years is the major reason for looking forward to retirement. However, after we retire, following an initial period of rest and relaxation, the prospect of endless leisure begins to feel almost oppressive. We begin to look forward to working again, not just because of the extra income but because of the significance that work gives to our lives.

Maintaining a positive balance between work and leisure was a near impossible task during our adult years. Now, however, the wisdom years offer us the chance to create and maintain such a balance.

In order to do so, we need to redefine both 'work' and 'leisure'. For me, work refers to the effort we invest in any large-scale project — the kind of activities that take up most of our time and demand most of our attention. In return, we hope to come up with a valuable result or end product, whether we are paid for it or not. According to this definition, writing this book is work — even though no salary was offered and the hours I have invested may not make financial sense.

Throughout this book I've been recommending that readers undertake their own individuation process. Using my definition, this process can most definitely be described as work — hard work, in fact.

During our adult years, the main purpose of work was to meet goals external to ourselves and our needs. During the wisdom years, we should strive to redirect this focus. The main meaning and purpose of work during this latest period of our lives is to build up our inner resources.

'Leisure' also needs to be redefined. It should not be limited to spending time lazing around the house. The commercial world is constantly trying to convince us to invest in various ways of escaping our work and daily lives, like vacation villages or ocean cruises. However, the leisure that comes with wisdom is the leisure to do the things we enjoy while nourishing mind, body and soul.

This kind of leisure includes the things you do when you take a break from work — like reading, watching TV or a movie, going for a walk or just chatting. It can also include activities like attending lectures, visiting museums or taking educational tours — edutainment. Anything you do which entertains you at the same time can enrich your life. Building ourselves up as people is not incompatible with spending time in quality leisure pursuits.

When our work and leisure combine, our everyday lives are enhanced. Having reached this level, we will be able to mindfully choose how to spend our time without feeling the need to escape from the seeming grind of daily life.

In achieving this synergy, you are likely to face a number of obstacles. Having retired, you may find that you need to go back to work just to make ends meet. Unfortunately, many of the jobs open to you will not make use of your full potential, nor at first glance give your life new purpose. However, you can find ways to enrich your inner life even in seemingly boring jobs by bringing your newfound inner wisdom to the fore.

For instance, if you end up working in customer service, observing the interaction between service providers and customers can be positive. You might well gain a better understanding of how people think and act in stressful situations, and even of what they can learn about themselves.

Aging and Illness

Aging is not a disease, nor a medical issue on its own.

On the one hand, as we progress through the aging process, we can expect more medical problems. These naturally lead to more interactions with the medical establishment, which will label you as an 'old person' naturally subject to a range of illnesses, suggest ways of coping with them and fill you with medications.

Allowing illness to overwhelm us detaches us from who we really are. This in turn detaches us from from the inner strength built up though our personal synergetic work and its positive influence on our health.

It is possible to adopt an alternative approach to coping with your growing physical weakness and associated problems. You should first harness the inner synergies you have developed, as this can be a powerful tool to delay physical deterioration.

Adopting this 'meta-medical' approach does not mean that you should ignore or neglect the importance of medical treatment, medication and hospitalization for your continued good health. There will be many cases where their help will be critical.

Here again you need to strike a balance between two complementary opposites. Aging without 'growing old' means knowing who you are and not becoming what you are told you should be. You should respect your doctor's opinions, but always submit them to the test of your critical self-awareness.

According to this holistic approach, being healthy means being content with life, despite your medical problems. If these problems narrow your horizons and undermine the things that give your life meaning, then you are ill indeed. On the other hand, if your curiosity and interests continue to widen despite the medical crises you may be facing, then you are still a healthy individual.

You can remain healthy if you can keep a balance between the things you are still able do and what you can't do any longer. Accepting your limitations while continuing to challenge them will lead you away from despair, from the temptation to give up on life and being overwhelmed by old age.

Our wisdom years will persist as long as we continue to make the effort to cope with the complementary contradictions of aging. Our spirit will continue to challenge the aging 'clock' even as the body weakens.

With a view to being an active observer of his own aging process, at the age of 88 psychoanalyst Samuel Atkin began keeping a personal, voice-recorded diary. He had been diagnosed with Parkinson's disease as well as vascular and heart disease. In addition, he suffered from the side effects of medications prescribed to control the progress of these diseases.

Despite these obstacles, Atkin continued to practice psychoanalysis until very close to his death. At the same time, his diary described his deteriorating health and his ever-increasing difficulties. He also documented his thoughts and feelings, his fluctuating moods and even his hallucinations.

Despite his failing body, Atkin made an effort to work a few hours each day, spurred on by the knowledge that he was still of use to his patients. 'In the past few years I have discovered that despite my fatigue and slower response there have been some positive qualitative changes in my work, undoubtedly a reflection of the inner changes in myself. I am bolder, more forthright in my interpretations ... . I have been observing, thinking, working, creating.'[3]

There is an essential qualitative difference between death at 70, for a person who has never experienced the benefits of the wisdom years, and death at the end of a long life in which these benefits were fully realized. The first is perceived as a troubling event; in the second case, we are able to make peace with the prospect of our imminent death.

If you have realized the wisdom years to the full, you can accept death with contentment and peace. At the end, this will grant you the ability to sum up your life from a positive perspective, leaving regrets behind. Death can also be viewed as part of the natural cycle of life. Being able to contemplate the next generation as a new link in the chain, a link which we had a part in creating, brings a sense of personal satisfaction.

The Roman emperor Marcus Aurelius (121–180 CE) was one of the more enlightened rulers in the history of humanity, as well as a leading Stoic philosopher. His book *Meditations: Thoughts to Myself*, written during his last years, was an early self-improvement manual. In the book, he suggests how we should take farewell of life: 'End thy journey in content, just as an olive falls off when it is ripe, blessing nature who produced it, and thanking the tree on which it grew.'[4]

Chapter 17

My Personal Journey

We each have our own journey to follow. Mine started over fifteen years ago. You may recall my surprise at receiving a formal letter from the Department of Social Security informing me of my eligibility for the old age pension (Chapter 1). The authorities were classifying me as old, while I felt that I was still in the prime of life. The surprise I felt led me to embark on a journey of reflection, research and personal experimentation, one which I've shared with you over the course of this book.

While the lessons to be learned are applicable to older people as a group, each of us is unique, meaning that we each should pave our own way on our journey of individuation. In this final chapter I want to tell the story of my own personal journey.

Following my initial surprise at being classified as old, the question of how many years I had left made me feel very anxious.

My family and personal medical histories were hardly encouraging. My father died of myocardial in-farction aged 47. My mother and my only sister had also died relatively young, after long and painful declines caused by dementia. For myself, I've been living with only one kidney since 1999, when the other one was removed due to cancer. In addition, like others in my family, I suffer from chronic high blood pressure. The odds of a long life are definitely stacked against me.

While most people can expect to live for a further ten years after retirement, it seemed unlikely that I could count myself among them. Naturally, I was extremely concerned at this prospect, and doubtful whether there was anything I could do about it. Thus motivated, I set out to analyze my chances of a longer lifespan and try to figure out a way to change what seemed like my fate.

While the prospects for enhancing my functional age seemed dire, the other dimensions of my make-up were much more positive. During my entire adult life I had dealt with complex social issues covering many fields. This experience had enabled me to develop advanced cognitive, mental and social skills.

I therefore decided that I would try to find out how to harness these positive characteristics in order to improve my physical state, if such a thing were possible.

Activating the Body

When I told my family physician that I was about to embark on a structured process aimed at enhancing my functional age she was very doubtful: 'I don't know of even a single piece of medical evidence which would indicate that what you want to achieve is possible. Just leave this nonsense alone.'

Although I had failed to convince her, I needed her co-operation, so I asked that she approve comprehensive quarterly blood and urine tests. These tests are simple and cheap, commonly used by family doctors for initial detection of changes in a patient's health. Comparing each quarter's results to previous tests would be a simple way of learning whether my physical health had deteriorated, remained stable or improved.

In addition, I signed up with a health club near my home, intending to use their facilities and classes rather than to undertake a physical training regime, which is what most members of such clubs want. I also wanted to train my body, but with a different goal in mind. My purpose was to become proficient at activating my body, so that I could achieve a synergy that would involve the four dimensions of my make-up simultaneously.

Of all the types of exercise offered at the club, I found that yoga and Pilates best served my purpose. My practice of both disciplines has improved the technique and quality of my breathing. I have acquired the skill of prolonging my inhalations and extending my exhalations throughout the length of my body.

This process enriches my brain with oxygen and improves its functioning. It also puts it in a state of cognitive and emotional alertness.

The focus on inhalations and exhalations means that my breathing in effect leads my body throughout the exercises. This transforms each session, and each time I feel a holistic enjoyment flood my body. I leave the class feeling a sense of empowerment and satisfaction. These feelings raise my spirits and improve my ability to cope with the issues and challenges which I face on a daily basis.

While exercising, I'm not in competition with other trainees, nor with myself. I focus solely on my breathing, its quality, and on performing each exercise as well as I can. I also strive to create an integrated flow of thought, emotion and movement while performing each pose.

At first, I had to concentrate on each pose separately. But, as I gained experience, I felt that I could relate to the whole series of exercises as one complete flow — just like life. Once I reached this level, I added power training sessions in order to maintain muscle mass and prevent loss of bone density. Unlike some other members of the club, I don't overexert myself, as developing a muscular body is the last thing that interests me.

During classes, I often deviate from the teachers' instructions and perform the exercises according to what feels right to me. The teachers and Instructors have learned to accept this behaviour with understanding and respect. Often, once class is over, they ask me to explain what motivates me and how I use the exercises to achieve my personal goals.

Even though I maintain my schedule at the gym rigorously, I don't consider myself an athlete or sportsman. I have no desire to become a marathon runner, a muscle-building freak or a yoga geek. I'm not addicted to the physical dimension of the training. Rather, I focus on the synergy of the physical with the cognitive, the emotional and the social, elements which act together to create an integrated personality.

Once I had mastered the exercises offered by the club, I created my own brief regime comprising a set of basic poses. I meticulously perform them every morning before I start my day. The daily repetition of the same exercises has become an enjoyable habit, providing both physical and mental satisfaction.

In addition to attending the health club, and my own daily exercise regime, a conscious awareness of how I activate my body has become an integral part of my daily routine. Whatever activity I do — walking, resting, sitting, typing, attending meetings or even washing dishes — becomes a springboard for awareness of my body and my breathing, and for the mindful appreciation of being in the here and now.

During my adult years, I regarded my body solely as a platform for other functions which I considered more important. Of course, I still get satisfaction from utilizing my body correctly. Beyond that, I've learned that this has important positive synergetic effects on the other elements of my make-up. In addition, I have gradually learned to apply the skills I acquired during physical training to other life situations. This has helped me cope better with everyday stresses and crises.

I've also learned to give more thought to the food I eat, without becoming a health-food freak. I'm not one of those people who follow vitamin, additive or dietary fads in the belief that doing so will delay the onset of old age. However, I have developed the ability to notice which foods make my body and mind feel good, and which don't. Consequently, I stay away from foods which don't have a positive effect on me, even if nutritionists recommend them.

I've also changed my attitude to the medical establishment. While I value and respect doctors and their recommendations, I don't accept them blindly. The same goes for the multitude of medications which they offer me as the answer to whatever problem I describe or as a preventative measure against future illness. I have also learned to question the need for medical tests, and to refuse those which I feel are redundant or even harmful.

The balance of power and responsibility between me as a patient and the medical establishment has changed. I'm no longer willing to accept that my opinion and judgment are irrelevant when the doctor gives his diagnosis and offers a suggested course of action. At the same time, I'm careful to examine each situation and issue on its own merits, assessing them in conjunction with the other lifestyle changes that I'm making.

Taking Small, Integrated Steps
for Positive Change

It is my belief that one should make many small, integrated adjustments, which together create meaningful change. These changes should be gradual and integrate with your existing lifestyle, your values and the skills you've already acquired.

I started on this course by selling my car — not an easy thing to do. In my former role as the owner of a company, my car was a status symbol. Initially, my friends perceived giving up the car as a reduction in status, implying a problem in the business. However, having sold the car, my status has been enhanced. These same worried friends now have even more respect for me and my company.

My friends were also doubtful whether I would manage to live without a car, assuming that it would limit my mobility. However, what happened was just the opposite. My mobility has not been reduced, while the transportation I use has increased in variety. I can get anywhere walking, riding my bike or using public transport. If none of these options are available, I can always take a cab. I've let go of the worries and tensions associated with driving on crowded roads and finding parking in town. A whole new world of new experiences, acquaintances and sensibilities has opened up for me. There are things you notice while biking which you don't when driving a car. There are also things you notice when walking which you won't see if you're riding a bicycle. Of course, this change has brought physical benefits as well, as I'm simply moving around more, rather than sitting in a car for hours.

I've also given up the position of CEO in the company I own, and have taken a back seat. Many of my friends also perceived this as a retreat, but the opposite is true. Stepping back became a step upwards, as it enabled me to create new avenues for activity within the company. My change in position helped me shake off old habits. This has proved to be a positive experience for me, as well as for my staff.

I also changed the way that my small but dedicated team of employees is remunerated. In addition to their level of responsibility and contribution to the company, we now consider the needs of their families. My own salary has been reduced, as I don't have as many financial obligations as before. I no longer need to support a family with young children, nor pay a mortgage. Since these duties are behind me, I wanted to do something to make life easier for the younger generation. Personally, I feel that I've gained a great deal from these changes and have not given up anything of real value.

I have also consciously modified and enriched my relationships with my significant others — spouse, family and friends. I now enjoy my time with them much more than in the past. I have found that my growing sensitivity to them has enriched my sensitivity to myself, as well as their understanding of me. In turn, this new attitude has also enhanced my ability to respond in a mindful and thoughtful manner to other people generally.

There are thus many situations where I now feel the positive effects of the integration of the emotional, logical, physical and social dimensions that the wisdom years offer us. The more I mindfully activate this integration, in whatever I am doing, the more fulfilling my life becomes.

During the overloaded period of adulthood, I got used to being a slave to the clock. I found myself in a never-ending chase to complete a task just to move on to the next one, without being fully present in either.

I've now learned to differentiate between what is significant to me and what is not, and rid myself of unnecessary time thieves. I try to do these meaningful activities slowly, focusing on the here and now and enjoying what I am doing.

I now intentionally make a point of doing everything I do without haste. According to conventional wisdom, slowing down is inevitable as we age. However, consciously slowing down is a choice which I had to learn and practise. Among its other benefits, it enables me to enjoy routine daily chores, like washing dishes, which I did not find enjoyable in the past. Slowing down is a good example of the integration between aging and a sense of purpose, enabling you to acquire new, meaningful and beneficial habits.

As a result of my new intentional approach to life, I have more time to think over what I am doing, both while I'm doing it and during what I call my 'time of reflection'. I do most of my reflecting at night, before I go to sleep, but also during weekends or relaxed walks which I take specifically for this purpose. During these times of reflection, I think about the meaning of recent events and my reactions at the time.

If I feel that I have let myself down in some way, I try to distinguish whether my failures were triggered by anger, disappointment or ego, or by the pursuit of respect, money or instant success.

These 'times of reflection' bring me a new and deeper understanding of events that I have been a part of. They also enable me to assume a more positive and relaxed frame of mind when I encounter similar situations in the future.

Everything I do teaches me lessons about the here and now, as well as causing me to rethink my personal goals and values. I find that the tangible and the abstract combine in my thoughts as the things that are happening in the moment interact with what I see as the deeper meaning in my life.

You may be wondering what happened to the long-range goal I had set for myself at the beginning of my journey. I was concerned to improve the dire state of my physical health, thereby increasing my life expectancy and helping me maintain quality of life in my later years.

Once I reached the age of 80, my doctor and I analyzed my health status by reviewing the results of my quarterly tests since the age of 67. The data validated what I felt in myself: there had been an improvement in some areas and no deterioration in others. Both were remarkable achievements, given that it's been thirteen years since the start of my journey. My doctor admitted that she was astonished at these results, which she could not explain by her knowledge of medical science alone.

This despite the deterioration in vision, hearing and memory which I have 'acquired' with old age.

My glaucoma is causing a gradual but significant deterioration in my sight and is putting me at risk of partial blindness. I will probably not be able to do without a hearing aid for much longer. My ability to remember names and dates, which has never been great, has also deteriorated.

However, none of these problems prevents me, in my 82nd year, from continuing to relish the mindful enjoyment of the wisdom years.

My chronological age advances with the relentless accuracy of a Swiss clock, one which seems to tick faster every year. Even so, I continue to enlarge the gap between my chronological age and my functional age — the only age which matters.

Although I'm getting older, I'm not yet old. In my 80s I could have found myself feeling and acting as a very old person. However, I feel, act and behave as though I am younger than many people in their 60s — even younger than I was during my 60s!

I increasingly forget names and dates, and my eyesight and hearing are poorer. However, I'm more aware of what goes on around me; I know how to ignore what is not necessary and focus on what's important to me. I give less value to general knowledge and rely more on my postformal wisdom. All in all, I'm more satisfied in my 80s than I was in my 60s.

I have taught myself to live in peace with the imperfection of aging, to find my own perfection within it and to accept the aging process that my body is experiencing. I have also learned to cherish the knowledge that, when the journey is over, I will be able to tell myself that it was all a great adventure.

I don't believe I'm boasting in saying this, even though this prospect gives me a certain measure of pride. I'm sharing my experience with you to assure you that you can reach this same goal, albeit in your own way.

Is the Wisdom Path for Everyone?

You may claim that my journey has been successful mainly due to the head start I enjoyed because of the professional interests I pursued during my working life. It is true that I have reached the wisdom years equipped with well-developed skills in the realms of thinking, emotion and social intelligence.

In addition, the transition from adulthood to later life has proved less traumatic for me than for many others. Since I own the company where I still work, I was never in a position to be fired or forced to retire, the kind of risks faced by most employees.

You may also question whether the various steps of the individuation process are effectively luxuries which can be afforded only by people who don't have economic problems which must be solved first.

This is the basic claim made by American psychologist Abraham Maslow in his celebrated hierarchy of needs, which assumes that each person has five basic needs in life.[1] For Maslow, proceeding though this hierarchy is like climbing a five-step ladder; only the satisfaction of the need expressed by the lower rung will enable the ascent to the next step. The first step represents physiological needs. The second step represents the need for safety. The third and fourth steps represent the need for social belonging and social esteem, respectively. Only having climbed so far can one proceed to the fifth and final step — self-actualization, or the need to harness one's entire suite of personal qualities in order to achieve self-fulfillment.[2]

According to Maslow's scheme, a person's basic existential, economic and security needs must be fulfilled before self-actualization becomes possible. In other words, if you have retired but lack adequate financial resources, you can't allow yourself the luxury of dealing with questions of self-development. Such deficits would automatically prevent you from entering the wisdom years.

Maslow's theory has been heavily criticized. I agree with those who claim that rather than being linear, people's needs are better regarded as concurrent. Even someone who struggles with their finances, and whose basic problem is making enough money to live, should not feel disqualified from enjoying the fruits of the wisdom years. Moreover, one of the benefits of the individuation process is that it can prepare you to find a job suitable for your needs, as well as providing personal satisfaction and personal growth.

In many respects, I accept that I do not represent the 'average' person. But does such a person even exist? I enjoy a number of advantages, but also experience disadvantages in life. You do, too. It is important that all of us seek to identify our weak points as well as our strengths. The next step is to integrate the various elements that make us who we are in order to overcome our deficits.

I would encourage each of you to adopt the approach to life presented in this book, and practise it in your own way. I firmly believe that following this path will start you on your personal voyage to claim the gift of the wisdom years.

Don't neglect the opportunity. You may miss out on the best time of your life.

References

Chapter 1 — Seeking a New Model of Aging

1. For the concept of perceptual relevance gaps, see Zvi Lanir, *Pinkas HaKis Shel Hashual* (*The Fox's Notebook*), an e-book published in Hebrew by Mendele Mocher Sfarim B'reshet, 2013. See esp. section 4, 'Why is the Summer Vacation during the Summer Vacation?'

2. According to the UN, a 65-year-old is considered old. See https://www.who.int/healthinfo/survey/ageingdefnolder/en.

3. See Zvi Lanir, *Fundamental Surprises* (Tel Aviv: Center for Strategic Studies, 1983).

4. On the concept of narrative identity, see https://en.wikipedia.org/wiki/narrative_identity.

Chapter 2 — Facing up to Retirement: Voices from the Street

1. All the names used in this chapter are fictional.

2. For further information on the concept of the 'fundamental crisis', see Lanir, *Fundamental Surprises*.

3. On the importance of conceptualization in these situations, see Lanir, *The Fox's Notebook*, esp. section 27, 'Teach yourself to Conceptualize'.

Chapter 3 — What can Economics and Demography Tell Us?

1. However, some scientists claim that life expectancy in the US has slowed in the past few years due to a national obesity epidemic.

2. See *World Population Ageing, 1950–2050* (Issue 207) (New York, NY: Population Division, DESA, United Nations, 2002).

3. See James Trefil, 'Can We Live Forever?', in *101 Things You Don't Know about Science and No One Else Does Either* (Boston, MA: Houghton Mifflin Harcourt, 1997), 211–16; Charles Q. Choi, 'Is There a Limit to the Human Life Span?', *Live Science*, 28 June 2017, https://www.livescience.com/59645-no-limit-to-human-life-span.html.

4. See E. M. Zelinski and R. F. Kennison, 'Not your Parents' Test Scores: Cohort Reduces Psychometric Aging Effects', *Psychology and Aging*, 22:3 (2007), 546–57, https://www.ncbi.nlm.nih.gov/pubmed/17874953 2007.

Chapter 4 — Asking the Experts: The Ladder Paradigm of Aging

1. See Patricia Sullivan, 'Gene D. Cohen, 65: Psychiatrist Broke Ground in Geriatrics', *The Washington Post*, 11 November 2009, http://www.washingtonpost.com/wp-dyn/content/article/2009/11/10/AR2009111018634.html?noredirect=on.

2. See Barbara Strauch, *The Secret Life of the Grown-up Brain: The Surprising Talents of the Middle-aged Mind* (New York: Viking, 2010), esp. chapter 7, 'Two Brains are Better than One'.

3. André Lemieux, 'Post-Formal Thought in Gerontagogy or Beyond Piaget', *Journal of Behavioral and Brain Science*, 2:3 (2012), 399–406.

4.	See https://harvardmagazine.com/2001/03/the-talent-for-aging-well-html.

5.	George E. Vaillant, *Triumphs of Experience — The Men of the Harvard Grant Study* (Cambridge, MA: Belknap Press of Harvard University Press, 2012).

6.	Ibid.

7.	Kuhn's groundbreaking study was first published as a book in 1962 by the University of Chicago Press; several new editions have since been published.

Chapter 5 — The Evolution of the Aging Brain

1.	The initial discoveries regarding the brain's emerging skills in later life were described by geriatric psychologists during the latter part of the twentieth century. Notable among them was Gene Cohen, a psychiatrist and geriatrician who was the first president of the Center on Aging, Health and Humanities at George Washington University and also worked at the US National Institute of Mental Health. He published several books on the subject, including *The Mature Mind: The Positive Power of the Aging Brain,* (New York, NY: Basic Books, 2006).

2.	Elkhonon Goldberg, *The Wisdom Paradox: How Your Mind Can Grow Stronger as Your Brain Grows Older* (New York, NY: Gotham Books, 2005).

3.	Ibid.

4.	See Kathleen Berger, *Invitation to the Life Span*, 2nd ed. (New York, NY: Worth Publishers, 2014), 399–401. See also https://en.wikipedia.org/wiki/Postformal_thought.

5.	See Daniel Kahneman, *Thinking, Fast and Slow* (New York, NY: Farrar, Straus & Giroux, 2011).

6. The concept of brain or mind maps is explored more fully in Chapter 6.

7. See Martin Lindauer, *Aging, Creativity and Art: A Positive Perspective on Late-life Development* (New York, NY: Springer, 2003).

8. See Ambar Chakravarty, 'The Creative Brain — Revisiting Concepts', *Medical Hypotheses*, 74:3 (2010), 606–12; Howard E. Gardner, *Art, Mind, and Brain: A Cognitive Approach to Creativity* (New York, NY: Basic Books, 1984); Edward De Bono, *Lateral Thinking: A Textbook of Creativity* (London: Penguin Books, 2009).

9. Gene D. Cohen, 'Research on Creativity and Aging: The Positive Impact of the Arts on Health and Illness', *Generations*, 30:1 (2006), 7–15, http://www. peopleandstories.net/wp-content/uploads/2011/08/ RESEARCH-ON-CREATIVITY-AND-AGING1.pdf.

10. See https://en.wikipedia.org/wiki/Creativity.

11. See Chakravarty, 'The Creative Brain'.

Chapter 6 — Creating New 'Mind Maps'

1. The term 'mind map' is also used for visual, hierarchical representations of concepts using words, images, symbols and signals. Mind maps are used as a tool for recording knowledge and model systems in learning, brainstorming and problem solving.

2. E. A. Maguire, K. Woollett and H. J. Spiers, 'London Taxi Drivers and Bus Drivers: A Structural MRI and Neuropsychological Analysis', *Hippocampus*, 16:12 (2006), 1091–101; K. Woollett and E. A. Maguire, 'Acquiring "the Knowledge" of London's Layout Drives Structural Brain Changes', *Current Biology*, 21:24 (2011), 2109–114.

3.   Norman Doidge, *The Brain That Changes Itself: Stories of Personal Triumph from the Frontiers of Brain Science* (New York, NY: Viking, 2007).

Chapter 8 — The First Hurdle: Ageism

1.   R. N. Butler, 'Age-ism: Another Form of Bigotry', *The Gerontologist*, 9:4 (1969), 243–46.

Chapter 9 — Understanding the Psychological Foundations of the Wisdom Years

1.   Jung died at the age of 83 (in 1961) after a brief illness. He was active and creative to the day of his death. In his own life, he showed that the process of individuation, accompanied by ongoing personal development, can continue until close to our deaths.

2.   See, for example, Vivian Diller, 'Midlife Crisis: A Myth or a Reality in Search of a New Name?', *Psychology Today*, 7 April 2011, https://www.psychologytoday.com/us/blog/face-it/201104/midlife-crisis-myth-or-reality-in-search-new-name.

3.   Margaret Mahler, *Separation–Individuation: The Selected Papers of Margaret S. Mahler*, Volume II (Northvale, NJ: J. Aronson, 1994).

4.   Peter Blos, 'The Second Individuation Process of Adolescence', *Psychoanalytic Study of the Child*, 22 (1967), 162–86.

Chapter 10 — How Our Brains Work: The Challenges Ahead

1.   These developments are described at length in Yuval Noah Harari's book, *Sapiens: A Brief History of Humankind* (London: Harvill Secker, 2014). I refer particularly to two central theses of his book. The first is that human history began 70,000 years ago with the

development of a distinctive form of awareness similar to that possessed by contemporary humans, and that it was this form of awareness which set in motion a new kind of cultural dynamics. The second is that since the linguistic revolution, people have lived in an 'imaginary order' — rules of thought and behaviour based on concepts that exist only in the common imagination of human beings: money, gods, justice, rights, nations, states and so on.

2.   See Kahneman, *Thinking, Fast and Slow*.

3.   I deal at length with the subject of changing habits in Part Three.

Chapter 11 — Renewing Mind and Body in Later Life

1.   Cognition refers to all actions related to the acquisition, processing and use of knowledge. The concept of cognition thus includes thinking, perception, understanding, learning, attention, creativity, reasoning, decision-making and problem-solving.

2.   See Deborah Danner, David Snowdon and Wallace Friesen, 'Positive Emotions in Early Life and Longevity: Findings from the Nun Study', *Journal of Personality and Social Psychology*, 80:5 (2001), 804–13.

3.   See Yaakov Stern, 'Cognitive Reserve', *Neuropsychologia*, 47:10 (2009), 2015–28. (2009), 2015–28.

4.   See Yaakov Stern, 'What is Cognitive Reserve? Theory and Research Application of the Reserve Concept', *Journal of the International Neuropsychological Society*, 8 (2002), 448–60, http://www.cumc.columbia.edu/dept/sergievsky/ pdfs/CogResTheory.pdf. See also Harvard Health Publishing, *What is Cognitive Reserve?*, https://www.health. harvard.edu/mind-and-mood/what-is-cognitive-reserve; Yaakov Stern, 'Cognitive Reserve in Ageing and Alzheimer's

Disease', *The Lancet Neurology*, 11:11 (2012), 1006–12.

5.   See Strauch, *The Secret Life of the Grown-up Brain*, Chapter 10, 'Brainpower Reserves'.

6.   For more on the difference between 'simple systems' and 'complex systems', see Lanir, *The Fox's Notebook*, section 16, 'The Fox and Thought as a Complex System'.

7.   Marian Rabinowitz, *The Six Ages of Man and the Inner Time* (Tel Aviv: Am Oved, 1985) [in Hebrew].

Chapter 12 — Mind Your Body

1.   See https://en.wikipedia.org/wiki/Brain-derived neurotrophic factor.

2.   On this subject, I have mostly followed Charles Duhigg, *The Power of Habit: Why we do what we do in Life and Business* (New York, NY: Random House, 2012).

3.   See Neil R. Carlson, *Physiology of Behavior*, 11th ed. (Boston, MA: Pearson, 2013). See also Gail Tripp and Jeff Wickens, 'Neurobiology of ADHD', *Neuropharmacology*, 57:7-8 (2009), 579–589; C. D. Fiorillo, P. N. Tobler and W. Schultz, 'Discrete Coding of Reward Probability and Uncertainty by Dopamine Neurons', *Science*, 299:5614 (2003), 1898–902.

Chapter 13 — Harnessing Our Brain Power

1.   Matthew Killingsworth and Daniel Gilbert, 'A Wandering Mind is an Unhappy Mind', *Science,* 330:6006 (2010), 932.

2.   For feelings seen as a cognitive activation lever (although differing from the present discussion), see Jim Davies, 'You Can Have Emotions you Don't Feel', *Nautilus*, 8 November 2016, http://nautil.us/blog/you-can-have-emotions-you-dont-feel.

3.	For the creation of concepts, and how they help us to create new knowledge, see Lanir, *The Fox's Notebook*.

Chapter 14 — Finding Happiness and Tackling Depression

1.	See Laura Carstensen, *Older People are Happier*, 2011, https://www.ted.com/talks/laura_carstensen_older_people_are_happier?language=en.

2.	See Deborah Netburn, 'The Aging Paradox: The Older we Get, the Happier we are', *Los Angeles Times*, 24 August 2016, http://www.latimes.com/science/sciencenow/la-sci-sn-older-people-happier-20160824-snap-story.html.

Chapter 15 — Resetting Relationships

1.	The author recognizes that his male perspective is limited. First published by Simon and Schuster in 1993, Betty Friedan's book *The Fountain of Age* offers a good description of such domestic phenomena from a feminine perspective.

2.	See further Lanir, *The Fox's Notebook*, esp. sections 18, 19 and 32.

3.	See Reuven Bar-On, 'The Bar-On Model of Emotional-social Intelligence (ESI)', *Psicothema*, 18:Suppl. (2006), 13–25.

4.	See Deeksha Sharma, 'Impact of Age on Emotional Intelligence and its Components', *International Journal of Research and Innovation in Social Science* (IJRISS), 1:1 (2017), 13–20.

5.	See Thomas M. Hess and Corinne Auman, 'Aging and Social Expertise: The Impact of Trait-Diagnostic Information on Impressions of Others', *Psychology and Aging*, 16:3 (2001), 497–510.

6.   Dan Buettner, *The Blue Zones: Lessons for Living Longer from the People who've Lived the Longest* (Washington, DC: National Geographic, 2008).

7.   In this chapter I have occasionally put the terms 'work' and 'retirement' in inverted commas. We need new terms to better reflect the new conditions of the wisdom years, but they are yet to be formulated.

8.   See Lawrence Kohlberg, *The Psychology of Moral Development: The Nature and Validity of Moral Stages*, Essays on Moral Development, vol. 2 (San Francisco, CA: Harper & Row, 1984).

Chapter 16 — Delaying Old Age

1.   Viktor Frankl, *The Unheard Cry for Meaning: Psychotherapy and Humanism* (New York, NY: Touchstone Simon & Schuster, 1978).

2.   *Optimal Experience: Psychological Studies of Flow in Consciousness*, eds Mihaly Csikszentmihalyi and Isabella Selega Csikszentmihalyi (Cambridge: Cambridge University Press, 1988).

3.   Betty Friedan includes these passages from Atkin in *The Fountain of Age* (New York, NY: Simon and Schuster, 1993), 250–53.

4.   Marcus Aurelius, *Meditations: Thoughts to Myself*, Book 4:48. The passage quoted is from *The Thoughts of the Emperor M. Aurelius Antonius*, trans. George Long (London: Bell and Daldy, 1862).

Chapter 17 — My Personal Journey

1.   For a summary of Maslow's schema, see Neel Burton, 'Our Hierarchy of Needs', *Psychology Today*, 23 May

2012, https://www.psychologytoday.com/us/blog/hide-and-seek/201205/our-hierarchy-needs.

2.   In his later years, Maslow added a sixth step, which represents the need for transcendence — giving oneself to something beyond oneself (such as the community involvement and volunteer work discussed in the present book).

Index

A

'active' thinking cycle *see* conscious thinking

adolescence, individuation 99

adulthood
appropriate goals 194
longest phase 75
moral development 189

aerobic exercise 140

age of wisdom *see* wisdom period

aged pension letter 9, 11, 207

ageism 79–89
raising awareness 82–83
UN recognition 82
workplace 80

aging
biological aspects 28–29
delaying decay 124
expressing love 172
and illness 203–206
mind maps 68
natural process 120
vs old age 193
power plant analogy 121–122
stereotypical reactions 80–81

aging population
burden of 34–35
growth rate 32–33, *33*

aloneness
dealing with 197–199
vs loneliness 197

Alzheimer's disease 117

antioxidants 144

anxiety thought stream 106

arborization
explained 64–65
illustrated *64*
London cabbies 67

assisted-living settings 25–26

Atkin, Samuel 205–206

attractiveness 181–182

avoidance 180–181

B

BDNF (brain-derived neurotrophic factor) 134

beauty stereotype 181–182

body
activating program 209–213
coping with decay 123
deterioration of 120–122

books, relationships with 182–183

brain
cell division 120–121
cooperation between lobes 110–113
improves with use 65–66
left hemisphere 108–110, 109–110
mature, new cells 118–119
neural network 63–64
new neurons 118–120
reward centre 136
right hemisphere 106–108, 109–110
structure of 103
synaptic connections *64*

brain functions, diminishing 49–53

'brain reserve', *vs* cognitive reserve 120

brain-derived neurotrophic factor (BDNF) 134

breathing
improved by exercise 210–211
mindful 166–169

Buettner, Dan 184

C

car
art of parking 112
decision to sell 214–215

CEO position, stepping down 215

change
conscious thinking 156–157
mobile phones 53
new habits 111–113
nutritional habits 143
positive steps 214–219
twenty-first century 10

childhood
  end of 75
  left brain 110
  preformal thinking 188–189
children, parents' expectations 174–175
chronological age vs functional age 35–36
cleverness vs wisdom 73
coffee, regular routine 145–146
cognitive reserve
  vs 'brain reserve' 120
  explained 117–118
community
  online 187–188
  sense of 185–186
computer games 142–143
concepts, logical process 111
conceptualization 154–156
conscious thinking
  explained 148–150
  feelings/senses 151–154
  new insight 154–156
  phase of change 156–157
coping skills 42–44
creativity
  from aloneness 197
  develops with age 60–61

D
dancing 143
data-processing speed 52–55
death
  accepting 206
  causes of 122
  start of 69
death certificate 122
denial, expressions of 12–13
depression
  causes for 168–169
  coping with 162–166
  medications 164
details, slower to grasp 52–53
diary, personal 205–206
discrimination 79–80
disputes 177

Doidge, Norman 68

E
emotional–social intelligence (ESI) 179
emotions, 'not logical' 110
Eric and Lara
  assisted-living 25–26
  zest for living 24–25
Erikson, Erik 96–98
Eriksson, Peter 118
ESI (emotional–social intelligence) 179
exercise
  aerobic 140
  improved breathing 210–211
  physical 133–134, 135
  power training 140–141
expectations
  need to meet 82
  of old age 81
  old age behaviour 86–87
  of parents 174–175
extended families, relationships 174–178

F
family relationships 174–178
feedback loop, cognition/neurology 115
feelings
  'not logical' 110
  vs sensing 151–153
'fight or flight' response 104–106
Follen, Michel 184
food, mindful approach 212–213
'formal thinking' 57
40-year-old crisis 97–98
Frankl, Viktor 195
Franklin, Benjamin 73
free radicals 144
freelancer, too hard 23–24
Freud, Sigmund
  internalization 81–82
  personality formation 93–94
friends/friendships 179–183

functional age
  vs chronological age 35–36
  explained 3–4
  factors determining 125, *125*

G
Goldberg, Elkhonon 56
Gould, Professor Elizabeth 118
grandchildren, interacting with 178
gym attendance 138

H
habit loop, McDonald's 136–137
habits
  eating 145
  forming new ones 134–139
  how to change 145
  need to change 111–113
  nutritional habits 143–146
  social avoidance 180–181
happiness
  described 159–160
  international study 150
  a new kind 160–162
Harvard Project on Aging 44–46
health
  family history 208
  old age 126–127
  quarterly review 218
hierarchy of needs 221–222
hippocampus, function 119
holidays, become boring 71–72
human organism *see* body

I
identity, loss of 16–17
illness and aging 203–206
imaginative abilities
  development of 107–108
  right to left hemispheres 109
individuation
  achieving 112–113
  benefits of 176–177, 181–182, 185, 222
  creative process 101
  effect on relationship 172–174

explained 94–96
mindfulness and 139–140
new mind maps 131
phases of 98–100
wisdom years 108
Industrial Revolution, workplace
  changes 75
infancy
  individuation 99
  right brain 109–110
internalization, process of 81–82
intuition 58–61
involvement without meddling 177

J
Jack, retirement experience 19–20
Jewish scriptures, cleverness *vs* wisdom 73
Jewish tradition
  boys' responsibility 75
  view of old age 86
Jung, Carl, personal growth theory 94–96

K
Kahneman, Professor Daniel 58
King Solomon 73
Kohlberg, Lawrence 188–189
Kuhn, Thomas 47

L
labour market, ageism in 80
ladder paradigm 40–42, *41*, 47–48
Lanir, Zvi (author), personal journey 207–222
left hemisphere (brain) 108–110
leisure, redefining 201–203
life expectancy
  21st century 36–37
  dramatic increase 2
  factors determining 125
  rising 31–33
life partner, seeing in a new way 172
life stages
  21st Century *76*
  new phase 74

traditional 74–75, 87–88
limitations, accepting 204–205
logic *vs* thought 43–44
London cabbies
   brain arborization 67
   skills requirements 66
loneliness 18–19
longevity 184–185
love, changing expression of 172
lung capacity 166–167

M
Marcus Aurelius 206
Maslow, Abraham 221–222
McDonald's, create habit loop 136–137
meaning of life, ongoing search 194–196
meddling 177
medical treatment, personal
   involvement 213
Meditations: Thoughts to Myself (book)
   206
memory, deterioration of 50–53
men, effect of retirement 173
'midlife crisis' 97–98
mind maps
   aging process 68
   cognitive connections 65
   individuation 131
   post-retirement 67–68
   work skills specific 67
mindfulness
   brain activation 156–157
   breathing 166–169
   coping with depression 165–166
   'here and now' 195–196
   household tasks 142
   learning 151–153
   for our bodies 139–140
mindset, creating new one 87
mobile phones, changing 53
'monkey thinking' 148, 150
mood swings 162–166
moral development 188–191

N
Nate, retirement experience 21–22
negativity 163–165
neurogenesis (brain cells) 118–119
neuron regeneration 144
Nun Study 115–117
nutritional habits, changing 143–146

O
old age
   vs aging 193
   conventional expectations 81
   current attitude 86–87
   factors determining health 126–127
   fighting against 19–20
   Jewish view 86
   pension letter 9, 11, 207
   reconciled to 19
   social stigma 79
   society's definition 79
'old age' market 81
'old' label 1
online communities 187–188
Orin, retirement experience 16–17
own company, enjoyment of 198–199

P
pension eligibility letter 9, 11, 207
personality formation 93–98
physical exercise 133–134, 135
physical weakness, growing 203–205
postformal thinking 57–58, 189–190
power plant analogy 121–122
power training 140–141
pre/postformal thinking 189–190
primal brain 104–106

R
Rabinowitz, Marian 126
reactive characteristics 105–106
'real' age 11
Reenie, retirement experience 17–19
relationships
   with books 182–183
   community 184–188

family 174–178
friends 179–183
intimate 171–174
modified and enriched 216
rebalancing 173–174
reptilian brain 104–106
retirees, view of 83–84
retirement
brain activation 113
effect on relationship 173
Freud's view 94
Jack's experience 19–20
Jung's view 94–96
ladder paradigm 40–42, *41*
mental vacuum 106
new freedom 72–73
old *vs* new view 88–89
Orin's experience 16–17
Reenie's experience 17–19
seeking information 29
right hemisphere (brain) 106–108,
109–110
routine 138–139

S
'scatterbrained', older people 55–56
security guard, older 22–24
self-employment, too hard 23–24
sensing *vs* feelings 151–153
separation, without detachment 176
shallow breathing 167
short-term memory 51–52
skills
declining 49–53
London cabbies 66
for older age 42–44
slowing down
consciously 216–217
grasping details 52–53
reflection time 54
social activism 186, 190
social attitudes 188–191
social avoidance 180–181
social expectations *see* expectations
social skills, increasing 179–180

'spiritual' identity 123–124
subconscious thinking 147–150
sugar addiction 145–146

T
The Brain that Changes Itself (book) 68
The Paradox of Wisdom (book) 56
The Structure of Scientific Revolutions
(book) 47
thinking, transforming 53–61
Thinking Fast and Slow (book) 58
thought *vs* logic 43–44
'time of reflection' 217–218
twenty-first century, change 10

V
vacations, become boring 71–72
Vaillant, George 45–46
vocabulary
'complimentary' terms 84
need new words 85–89
positive veneer 84
volunteers 186 187

W
wisdom period
individuation 99–100, 108
losses during 193–194
new life stage 76–77
source of term 73
transition stage 2–3
wisdom *vs* cleverness 73
women, effect of retirement 173
work
redefining 200–203
return to 21–22, 59, 202–203
'working' memory 51–52
workplace, ageism in 80

Y
yoga 138–139
youth, modern roles 77

Z
zest for living 24–25